IT TAKES GUTS

A story of love,
hope and a missing bowel

Thank you for saving lives

IT TAKES GUTS

First published in 2014 by
Panoma Press

48 St Vincent Drive, St Albans, Herts, AL1 5SJ, UK

info@panomapress.com
www.panomapress.com

Book layout by Charlotte Mouncey
Printed on acid-free paper from managed forests.

ISBN 978-1-909623-72-9

The right of Evelyne Brink to be identified as the author of this work has been asserted in accordance with sections 77 and 78 of the Copyright Designs and Patents Act 1988.

A CIP catalogue record for this book is available from the British Library.

All rights reserved. No part of this book may be reproduced in any material form (including photocopying or storing in any medium by electronic means and whether or not transiently or incidentally to some other use of this publication) without the written permission of the copyright holder except in accordance with the provisions of the Copyright, Design and Patents Act 1988. Applications for the Copyright holders written permission to reproduce any part of this publication should be addressed to the publishers.

This book is available online and in bookstores.

Copyright 2014 Evelyne Brink

IT TAKES GUTS

A story of love,
hope and a missing bowel

Evelyne Brink

Praise For 'It Takes Guts'

"An amazing story of how crisis can turn strangers into family and the amazing reserves of grace, love, and hope we can all find inside ourselves when we really need them."

Michael Neill, author of Supercoach, The Inside Out Revolution and Founder of Supercoach Academy

"This story will make you weep and laugh. It will make you feel every feeling there is – and think deeply about what is real, sacred and true about life."

Robert Holden, author Holy Shift! and Founder of The Happiness Project

"If you want to quickly reduce the size of almost any huge problem you are dealing with, simply read *It Takes Guts* by Evelyne Brink."

Steve Hardison, The Ultimate coach

"Evelyne and Tuffel's story will inspire you – it will make you smile and it will also make you weep. Hang on for the ride because there is much this brave boy and his mother have to teach us all about the extraordinary nature of life."

Rich Litvin, author of "The Prosperous Coach" and founder of the Confident Woman's Salon.

"This is a truly powerful story that can and will change the world. The amount of humour, absolute love, raw humanness and shifts in perspective in this short book have altered my view of what I think is possible. Thank you

Tuffel for your light and wisdom; I am forever brightened by your story."

Amy Deva, Intuitive coach and yoga teacher

"Wow – Evelyne's story is so in heartfelt and touching to my core. I too had a baby that was hospitalized in intensive care and was told he would not survive. I felt like Evelyne was telling my story and what I personally went through from the strength she had to have to stand up for her baby to the constant looking for every bright side. Her story brought tears of joy and tears of empathy in knowing the power it takes to believe in your baby and in miracles within the universe. I am in awe of the complete connection Evelyne, Thomas and Tuffel have to change their circumstances – and in doing so, the world."

Darlene Navarre, Playologist, Founder of GoPlazy

"*It Takes Guts* is raw, real and deeply moving. It gets you in sync with the power of human emotion and how capable we are of creating miracles when we believe in nothing less. I am in awe of this book."

Marilyn Rodriguez,
Founder, Embrace Your Light Coaching

CONTENTS

Praise For *'It Takes Guts"*	5
Forewords	11
Introduction	15
CHAPTER 1 Life will never be the same (oh, and it's a boy) January 2012	17
CHAPTER 2 Life with the Tuffelmeister (3 weeks later)	29
CHAPTER 3 Tuffel and the joys of motherhood (1.5 months)	39
CHAPTER 4 Life is sweet. Sometimes. (2.5 months)	47
CHAPTER 5 The art of empowerment or how to save a baby from the operating table (Tuffel is now 3 months old)	61
CHAPTER 6 Prince Tuffel at King's Hospital from surviving to thriving (4 months)	71
CHAPTER 7 Are you ready for another miracle? (4 months)	81

CHAPTER 8 — 87
Amazing Grace
(4 months)

CHAPTER 9 — 93
We could all use a lesson in self-soothing
(4 months)

CHAPTER 10 — 105
Oh, such a perfect day
(5 months)

CHAPTER 11 — 111
All change! Wards, tubes and moods
(6 months)

CHAPTER 12 — 119
Coping and hoping
(6 months)

CHAPTER 13: — 129
Life at Evelina Children's Hospital
(6 months)

CHAPTER 14 — 137
There is no place like... Can I please go now?
(7 months)

CHAPTER 15 — 151
Holiday... Celebrate!
(8 months)

CHAPTER 16 — 157
Trust your gut
(9 months)

CHAPTER 17   163
Everybody needs a Bridget
(8 months)

CHAPTER 18   171
Opening up
(10 months)

CHAPTER 19   177
How to make a miracle
(10 months)

CHAPTER 20   183
Christmas gagagadada style
(11 months)

CHAPTER 21   189
Happy Birthday!

CHAPTER 22   193
The big One
(12 months)

Epilogue   197

Thank Yous   201

Further Reading   205

About the Author   207

Forewords

Fact is stranger than fiction and you would be forgiven for believing that a lot of this story is made up – but it isn't! Tuffel really is a special, almost unique, baby, and he and his family have experienced challenges that fortunately very few of us ever face. I often wonder how I would cope with any particular adversity, and part of the beauty of this book is that Evelyne is showing one way how. Another part is the actual story!

Another quality of the book is the insight it gives you into who Evelyne is. What you read here is what you get! I can vouch for many of the details for the first five months since I witnessed them. That does not include Evelyne's secret fantasies revolving around uniforms!

It was impossible not to feel very involved in this story. It provoked many reactions as I read on. First of all, amazement at all Evelyne went through physically – even though I witnessed a small portion of it. Second: amazement at what she went through emotionally – I don't recall seeing any of that! Third: amusement because of the light-hearted way she has expressed what the family went through. Fourth: interest in the style and organisation of her writing; I am sure I would have been much more turgid if I had tried to do it. Fifth: gratitude. She has helped me a little bit to understand the experience of patients and families. I say a little bit because I would not be so presumptuous to claim I could feel her experiences. Finally, I didn't want the book to finish where it did – I wanted it to go on to its ultimate happy ending....

As a Neonatal Unit consultant, I (like most of my colleagues) have never experienced neonatal intensive care first hand. To have the opportunity to find out how the babies and their families are experiencing our care is beyond price. Evelyne succeeds in drawing this picture and involving us in how it affected Tuffel, Thomas and herself. These effects will be life long. And of course, the story is not yet finished…

A M Kaiser

Anthony Kaiser BSc MD FRCP FRCPCH

Consultant neonatologist

St Thomas' Hospital, London

Evelyne Brink is an extraordinary woman. An incredible performer – once Europe's most successful Madonna impersonator – she's now a highly respected personal and executive coach.

She was pregnant and counting down the days to becoming a mother for the first time, when on the very day that was supposed to be the happiest of her life, her whole world seemed to screech to a blood-curdling halt.

Within minutes of giving birth to a beautiful blue-eyed baby boy, she was told the worst news a mother could ever hear: "Your baby is going to die."

But Evelyne is a coach. She has a career based on helping people undertake the 'impossible' on a regular basis, and teaching them to break through 'impossible' barriers.

And she wasn't ready to hear this heartbreaking news.

So she gathered up her courage and she stepped up in an incredible way.

I was privileged to spend time in hospital with her son Tuffel when he was four months old. He was strapped to several beeping machines; cords and cables ran into and out of his body. But he was alive. And he was thriving.

Evelyne had refused to accept the doctors' prognosis when he was born and here we were, watching her lovely baby rolling from his back to his tummy.

Tuffel is now two years old and the journey hasn't always been an easy one. There have been midnight blue-light ambulance trips to the hospital and scares and challenges.

But Evelyne has shown up with heart and soul throughout. And until now she's shared this only with her private clients and the readers of her blog.

There is hope that stem cell research will offer a brighter future. But Evelyne still takes the journey one day at a time. The only way we can ever really live life.

Evelyne and Tuffel's story will inspire you – it will make you smile and it will also make you weep. Hang on for the ride because there is much this brave boy and his mother have to teach us all about the extraordinary nature of life.

Rich Litvin

Rich Litvin,
Founder of The Confident Woman's Salon
Los Angeles, March 2014

Introduction

Meet my son Tuffel: when he was born, we were told he wouldn't survive.

His small intestine completely destroyed, he'd be unable to absorb food. Ever. Hundreds of people around the world have lit candles, sending wishes and prayers. About 50 outstanding nurses and two handfuls of incredible doctors have been looking after him, day and night. Believing in better, we have put our minds together to create solutions out of the ordinary.

This is his story and ours, through our first year of miracles. He has been thriving against the odds, teaching us about living in the now and the power of love, humour and sterile gloves.

PS: The people, places and occurrences in this book are real. Some names have been changed for privacy (when I didn't have a way to gain permission) and this has been noted. No animals were harmed in the making of this book, except the bacteria we regularly defeat with disinfectants.

CHAPTER 1

Life will never be the same (oh, and it's a boy)

JANUARY 2012

He's here. Every day is a gift...

I'd wanted to send one of those text message round-robins written hastily before the chaos of new-baby reality breaks loose:

> *Dear friends,*
>
> *Our son Tuffel was born on Friday,*
> *January 20th at 2:15am weighing 2.86 kg*
> *(6.3 pounds or so). Labour was short*
> *and sweet and we are all ever so well*
> *and happy.*
>
> *Love, Evelyne*

But in my life things seem to be a little different. Here is the version I would have to send instead:

> *Dear friends:*
>
> *Our son Tuffel was born on Friday,*
> *January 20th at 2:15am. Labour was*
> *induced due to a medical condition –*

a prognosed bowel obstruction – and took 36 hours.

I don't want to listen to my relaxation playlist EVER again. I know too well when the next bloody bird chirps through the waterfall. When you can sing along to Stream of Dreams Nature Sounds Volume 2, *things have clearly gone too far.*

I managed without painkillers except for a bit of gas and air in between (after 32 hours or so).

Tuffel weighs 2.86kg and looks healthy. But he is not.

He was operated on, at only 12 hours old. Within his first 24 hours, he was sentenced to death.

We were told that his small intestines were completely destroyed and he wouldn't be able to live.

He is a strong boy with fair hair (hint of ginger) and blue eyes. He is extremely cute and serene. All other organs are perfectly fine. He is just missing the bowel. Without which, one cannot process food.

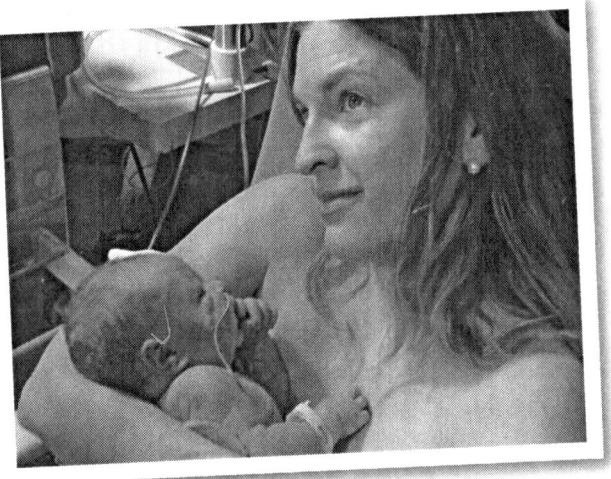

Sometimes life is shit. We all know that. Sometimes shit hits the fan. It's messy, sure. But you know what, we would love that right now. Because in our case there is no shit. And *that* is a much bigger problem!

- Apparently bowels don't really grow much
- A healthy adult has around six metres of bowel; anything less than two metres is classified as Short Bowel Syndrome (SBS)
- Even babies born with a short bowel usually have 50cms
- Ours has less than 10cm
- Bowels are the hardest organs to transplant
- Bowels are the most complex organ in the body

So much for our family dream...

Nine months of hardcore pregnancy with immobility and pains, and when the doctors had discovered a cyst in week 20, well, that wasn't fun. I'll be honest with you, that's when my plan to write a funny book on pregnancy came to a halt. *From Yummy To Mummy – a humorous journey into motherhood* had sounded like such a good idea at the time, but I doubted that what was happening to me was really what first-timer 'preggeratis' would like to read about.

But they had said it was quite common. The cyst. It goes or they take it out. Simple. But things had gone to worse from there. Just when I had my optimism back at 30 weeks, they saw some loops of bowel floating and offered four case scenarios for us:

1. Cystic fibrosis
2. Down's Syndrome
3. Bowel obstruction
4. We got it wrong

We had wished for option 4, with option 3 as plan B. The bowel obstruction. After genetic testing, the medics seemed to settle on this diagnosis and prepared us for a stay in hospital of up to three months. I had been devastated. But three months was the worst case scenario.

And now, after two days and two nights of very challenging medically induced labour (far removed from my home water birthing idea), this?

"We're sorry but I don't think he's going to make it."

"Is there not a tiny bit of hope?" I had probed. Their eyes told me what I didn't want to hear. "Well there is always a bit of hope I suppose."

"Then we take that bit of hope and we build it from there." I was determined. That was my initiation to motherhood.

"And even if he'd make it through, we are talking two to four years in hospital initially." That's not really what I call a best-case scenario, but as we know, everything in life is relative.

We'd already suffered through a painful miscarriage that had landed me in hospital on morphine the previous March. Surely nobody deserves such bad luck? This is wrong!

I'm a personal and executive coach – I help people to be happier and more successful, and look at my life!

Ever since my partner Thomas and I started studying the psychology of happiness, we've been dealing with the toughest challenges (i.e I nearly lost him in Peru when he got severely ill in the mountains) and counting. This is so surreal. I discharged myself from hospital the same day – no way I'd let Thomas sleep alone at home – and have been back and forth since then. We need a miracle. A pretty big one.

Fast forward to Monday – you don't have to relive this weekend with me (the pain and the tears with our distraught families) – we met Dr Jonathan Hind, Consultant in Paediatric Hepatology, Intestinal Rehabilitation and Transplantation – in short, the specialist consultant from King's College Hospital who knows about bowels and the lack thereof.

I don't know how often you've time travelled or felt like the film you were watching was suddenly swapped with another one, but it felt as if a whole different slide show had been inserted into the projector: Doctor Hind said there was a chance that Tuffel could live on a form of artificial nutrition called Total Parenteral Nutrition (TPN), which is given intravenously, and due to recent medical advances doesn't necessarily destroy the liver as it used to.

Miracle number one! There is hope!

However, life on a drip is challenging to say the least. Infections are a constant threat to life, as is the possibility of veins closing up. We'd live on borrowed time, in a way. Transplants still have high mortality rates, but again, due to medicine advancing so fast, they are becoming more common. Plus, new immunosuppressant drugs are being developed that kill fewer people .

At this point, all we know is that immune suppression isn't funny because living without an immune system means having to take a lot of drugs to guard against any kind of infections, colds and what have you. Not to mention that immunosuppressive drugs have side effects – one of which is cancer. We also know that transplant survival is not a given. We understand that the battle for our new child could be an ongoing one.

"And one of you will have to give up work. This is a full-time job. There will be alarms going off throughout the night and ongoing things to be sorted. You will be tired and very busy looking after him," concluded the consultant, nodding his head.

Thomas looked at me. It was clear the family would from now on rely on him to bring in the bacon and he was just in the process of starting up a business.

"Well," I countered. "Lucky I don't have a normal job. I can still write books, can't I?" The thought of a book tour comes to mind and painfully pops. How would I ever travel with a child reliant on machines?

What will happen to all my dreams of being an inspirational speaker, coach and author jetting around the world sharing grounded ways of freeing oneself up to live a wonderful life? I see myself delivering seminars, workshops and personal coaching sessions to people who want to create a meaningful legacy. The last few years have seen me establish my international coaching practice, and may I say, quite successfully. All that would now be in vain? Really? My life would boil down to being a carer to a disabled child? Is that what we're talking about? I once had a glamorous career and the opportunity to be part of society in this way would be taken from me just like that?

I stopped myself in my tracks. This wasn't about me. This was about our child. But 'our child' was a very new situation for us.

I'd heard before that once you have children, they come first. To be honest, that was also my a secret fear – I know many women struggle with the question of who they are once they become mums and everything changes. I have a strong sense of who I am and what I want to do in my life. I've also always desired a loving family. My determination has always been to bring the two together – in fact, I believe that they belong together. This idea was being shattered as I learned that our best chance meant putting myself last and this little bundle first.

What was to become of life? Is that what they mean when they say everything changes once you have baby? Admittedly, this is not really what I signed up for. I wasn't asked. As much as I'd learned in coaching to create your wonderful life and achieve goals and do what you love, following your heart, some things are just not in our power. And they may be the biggest things. This was a deeply humbling and uncomfortable lesson.

Curiously, once I shifted my focus away from my personal woes, I felt lighter and more at ease in this strange situation. I wasn't really willing to judge it too much or give it too much meaning as a strong sense of unknowing paired with a sense of possibility expanded inside me. Who knows where life would take us from here? Who knows what adventures would lie ahead? Who knows what miracles could potentially unfold?

Nobody can tell me what I'm able to do – or not do. Nobody knows what this little man will be able to do, or not do. From what we understood this was a rare and relatively unknown situation. We needed to believe in the possibilities without getting caught up in them. Leave expectations by the wayside and become fully present in the moment. This is the space in which miracles happen. I had studied that and now was the time to put it to the test. A test I really hoped not to fail, but didn't allow myself to think through too much. I don't have to go where the pain lives. I'm okay in the now.

To give you an idea of how rare our situation is, although there are some support groups for TPN families in the US, we were told there are none here in the UK. There are only a few cases, and we're trying to track them down so we can connect. We need to speak with others who know about this. There must be someone somewhere!

We don't know what will become of our little one. We are thrown into a lifelong uncertainty and don't know what lifelong even means for him. For now, he is in the Intensive Care Unit – well, actually, he's moved to High Dependency because he recovered so well from surgery. Yes, little Tuffel is already moving up in the world.

He's got two tubes running to his tummy through his nose, a line in his arm for food, another line from his tummy and a big scar from being cut open. He is extremely cute and everyone is falling in love with him – so beware. When I held him in my arms, it was the most amazing and the most heartbreaking experience of my life. His little blue eyes have seen mine full of tears too much already. They are so pure, so clear, so calm.

He's a Zen master but he's also quite a cheeky chappy. When being X-rayed, he peed all over the table in one high bow, wetting the equipment and nurses. Now *that's* my boy! He managed to take off his mittens (which he wears to prevent him from pulling on the tubes) and rip out the tubes the nurse spent all day inserting. We need the tubes to drain whatever is in the stomach and top bowel so that it can deflate and heal, then we can see what we've actually really got left. Every centimetre will count. We really want him to grow some bowel. More than they say is possible. Insert miracle here. Please.

There are some relatively new procedures to lengthen and stretch the bowel, but only if we have some! We really make it convenient for God to find good use of his miracle time. He just needs to pop by the Neonatal Unit at St Thomas' Hospital (Tuffel is in Room 2). There are plenty of opportunities for miracles and very happy receivers.

However, in all this despair and sadness, beauty is unfolding. Thomas' parents flew in from Denmark; my 93-year-old great aunt left her flat to come to the hospital; my mother is here and family and friends gather closer than ever.

A global research and support team has formed – I'll call it Team Tuffel. With agents in China (my sister is currently there with her six-month old), Germany (where my mother still lives), Lanzarote (Dad is on holiday there, but still pulling his strings from an island with less reception than the Tundra in Russia). We have Denmark on the case and America. The US is the most advanced with the new procedures, and my family there (I was an exchange student when I was 16) is connecting us with the top bowel specialist in the country, spending hours on research and networking for us. Our American friends we met on a trip to South America are helping too, as well as our family in the UK. It's incredible. Just incredible. I am soothed in a net of love and support.

We have churches in the UK and US praying for him, healing light being sent from Berlin. Candles are being lit in various places thanks to the Hypnobirthing community,

I just heard. Friends, mates, and even people I don't know tell me they send prayers and let other people know to send divine thoughts and love our way. I do believe that makes a difference. Feeling the connections where they weren't before makes me all warm and fuzzy.

Tuffel – we made up his name and also the meaning. It's now a registered name in the UK and in a German passport and it stands for 'he who is endlessly loved and cared for, has a strong will to live and a wicked sense of humour.' Let's see what this little boy holds in store for us.

I had a deep conversation with renowned transformative coach Michael Neill yesterday about the difference between experiencing life as a rollercoaster or a river. *(Michael has been my personal coach and generously sprang to action when he heard my news offering his time to help me connect to my wellbeing in this crazy situation)* He reminded me that if we evaluate life from the level of our moment-by-moment experiences, we live as if we are going up and down on a rollercoaster. (Yeah, tell me about it!) When we see that there is life beyond our individual experience – or when we sense the current of energy that's always flowing in the background and that we just happen to be part of – we can feel a deep sense of peace and wellbeing as we bob along on that 'river of life'. We don't control the river; we don't know what's coming. But if we can trust that we are a part of the river, new possibilities and resources within us begin to emerge as the journey unfolds.

So I'm letting life take me where I need to go. And it makes me feel incredibly peaceful to think of myself being of the river rather than trying to desperately hang onto something.

The prayers and thoughts and research efforts are all part of an incredible energy that I do believe Tuffel will sense. I'm just in awe of it all. Humbled by the amount of love and care.

My invitation for you is to join me in the space of possibilities. We are all from that same amazing energy and have the potential to create outstanding lives for ourselves and others. What will you do with your gift called life and health today?

I'll take mine to the hospital and cuddle and love my little boy. Sing to him hours on end, get him onto my bare chest, stroke him and soothe him with my little finger, which he loves to suck.

CHAPTER 2
Life with the Tuffelmeister
(3 WEEKS LATER)

It has only been three weeks since the birth of little T and my life has drastically changed. Of course it was going to anyway, but all the devastating news of his condition topped the expectations and shocked even our doctors. And I'm not talking about junior docs, but the crème de la crème of paediatric consultants.

I've been so grateful for the prayers, candles, thoughts and good wishes that have come our way. These have extended to Spain, Australia and Israel – wow.

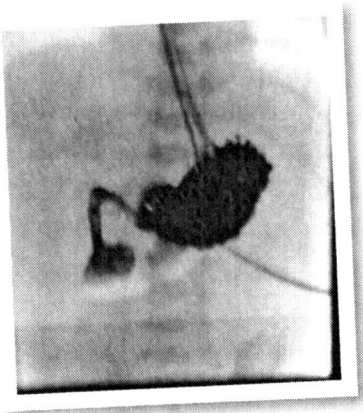

The image here shows the X-ray of his contrast study, which reveals just how much bowel we've got to work with. We knew there might be seven to 10 centimetres and now we know what it really is. The total amounts to zero.

Absolutely nothing. Which means Tuffel won't be able to process food. Ever. A life on artificial nutrition, intravenously fed. Here you see the stomach with the little bit of duodenum (the first section of the small intestine that adds juice from the gallbladder but doesn't really break down or absorb food).

To give an idea of size, the stomach is as big as a walnut.

Yes, we were rather taken aback by the result. We had so hoped for more and yet, got less…Time for more tears and giving up hope? Never!

When you look at a cloud, you will have a very different experience from being in the cloud. Living with Tuffel is a very different experience from the snapshot of his 'story'. The story sounds so final, but life keeps flowing. So I'd like to share about some of that life.

The human brain is incredibly adaptable. So for us, the strange fact that our baby isn't at home in the evening, that I sit all day with him in a ward with five other babies in the 'high dependency' unit of the Neonatal Ward – that's normal. It's *my* norm. The beeping of the machines, the tubes, the lines, the little plastic see-through cot that looks like a washing basket. The little bags with green stuff hanging off my son.

We don't know anything different.

I'll admit, it doesn't feel normal when I write it all down. I can see how having a baby on strings isn't normal: I have seen enough babies to know.

Thomas and I took a break and went on a walk the other day. We crossed Westminster Bridge and wandered all the way to Covent Garden. Being amongst 'normal' people in London, walking past and into shops was a highly surreal experience. And I was reminded that some people have mobile babies. Wireless infants they push around in chairs with wheels on that aren't wheelchairs. Fascinating.

And it does take mental effort to not get jealous and think: 'I should have one of those!' I have a wired baby, tied to a hospital corner. But then again, the corner of St. Thomas' hospital that we are tied to happens to be one of the most beautiful spots in London with views of the Thames and the London Eye, so I can't complain.

Living in HDU (the High Dependency Unit) is a world of its own. The nurses change daily. With one nurse for two babies, there are three in the room most of the time. We are so well taken care of. My respect for nurses has soared: I proclaim them to be the world's most undervalued superheroes. Apart from the work they do administering medicines, they are being strong for us, too: giving me space to shed a tear, talk or share a joke. From my once-imagined future as a stay-at-home-mum – sitting at home working, writing, coaching, and dreading the ceiling falling on my head – I'm now part of an active social hub. A very private members' club I never applied for. It has a rather limited drinking licence (tea and coffee, I'm afraid) but it makes up for this by sporting a microwave in the Green Room and it's very exclusive indeed. Besides, you couldn't afford the membership fees if you tried!

Our room has blue walls and neon lights. Six cots. Monitors everywhere. Under Tuffel's cot is a little cupboard, where I store some clothes, nappies and my most valued accessory: the breastfeeding pillow. I can't breastfeed, but it's invaluable for sitting with Tuffy.

Tuffel's nose and cheek are taped up to keep his tube in place. He looks somewhere between sweet and sorry, depending on how well it's taped.

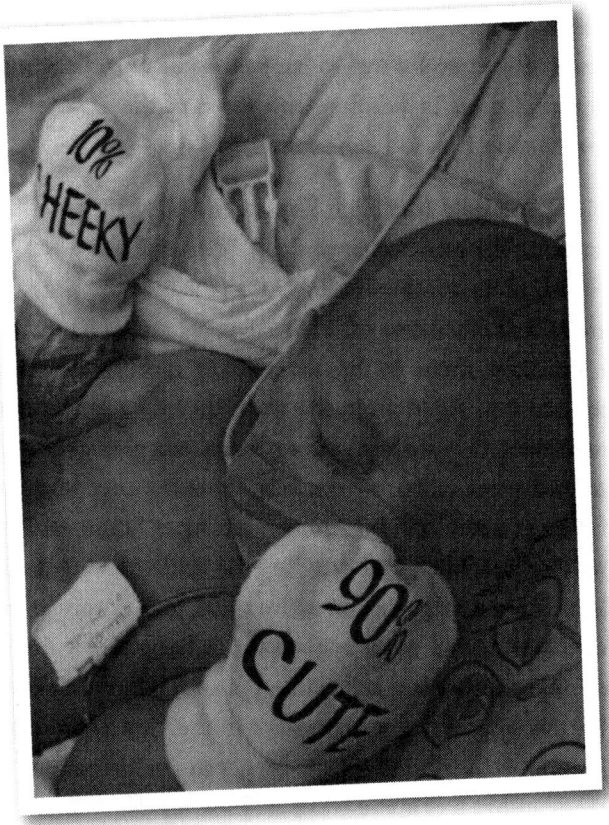

Of course, he loves pulling at the wires, but it takes half a day and lots of discomfort to insert a tube like that, so you can imagine I go into mama-hawk mode watching over this. When I am not there, he gets to wear mittens, which look like cotton boxing gloves, and is restrained in a white blanket. It's a kind of baby fetish called swaddling and, luckily, babies like it. How did they find out about it? Did someone tie up their baby in various ways and discover that chains, handcuffs and ropes aren't so favourable but a blanket-mummifying procedure tested popular? Some things we will never know…

He has a line going into his vein, through which he gets fed the white space food called TPN (Total Parenteral Nutrition – doesn't it read like 'parental'? It's not; it's para enteral, going past the digestive tract. A bit like paranormal but less woo-woo). The tube coming out of his tummy with a bag attached, which takes out his stomach contents (waste products of the TPN, plus saliva), I call the Teletubby Tube. There is also a little opening next to it (covered in a clean dressing) that allows a tube to be inserted, which goes into the lower part of the bowel (the colon). It looks like another belly button, except it's red.

A few days ago, he had a cannula fitted in his little head to insert antibiotics, as he was going through his first infection. He sported a little plastic container on it, stupidly designed like a small yogurt pot. Apparently it helps prevent him from shaking or pulling out the cannula. If you put a yoghurt pot on my head I'd do far worse things than pulling...

So, life with Tuffy... I sit there and hold him. I take him out of the crib, which involves holding onto the two or three bags, the attached lines and the drip lines that all tangle up no matter how you do it. Doctors, nurses, surgeons come along and probe him at various times of the day. For that we put him back to the crib and try to detangle his lines and bags.

Heel pricking for blood tests follow. Listening to his heartbeat. Changing the dressing on the opening on his stomach. Emptying out the little bags. Replenishing the fluids that run through the drips. Inserting medicines when needed. X-raying where needed to see if a tube is in the right place. All sorts of annoyances this little fellow has to endure before he gets the real pleasure of having his nappy changed and weeing all over the place like a proper little boy.

But – as tragic as not having a small bowel is – he never smells bad, as there is no poo. We have to see the good in everything. I admire this little man and how calm he is throughout all he's going through. He is a gutsy little boy – even though he has no gut.

Despite being well nourished, the stomach, being empty, still sends out hunger signals to the brain. And seeing him wanting my breast, opening his mouth, sometimes screaming and shaking his head, arching his back – all signs of "I AM FREAKING HUNGRYYYY" – that really gets to me. I've got the breast, I've got the milk, I get the signs and there is nothing I can do about it.

I feel so helpless.

I am not allowed to feed as we can't allow milk to linger in the cul de sac of his duodenum. Sometimes I cry alongside my son; it hurts not to attend to his need. But most of the time I just sit there with my top off, my engorged bosom for all to see, and cuddle him. I hardly have to wash my tops anymore as I don't wear any during the day. Apparently, new mums look a mess with sick on their clothes and milk seeping through. Being topless completely solves that problem, people. Lucky it's warm in the unit. Skin-to-skin care is the best for baby and definitely for mummy. Shame and decency go right out the window (where they belong).

I am busy holding my son. Every 3.5 hours I add a breast pump to complete the look. Hospital breast pumps are the Rottweilers of breast pumps. The one I use is so strong it sticks to my breast (look mummy, no hands!) whilst mauling my nipples, extracting the 'gold dust' (aka breast milk). More of where that goes later…

Tuffel also loves sucking on my finger (or Daddy's, for that matter). That's his favourite soother. It feels like he's sucking our fingers off – they get all white and soft after a while. But I'll happily give my finger – it's the closest he's getting to a breast. It feels like we are cheating him a bit, but that's the best we can do right now.

Our music choice: Mozart. Tuffy has his little MP3 player and mini speaker we use to blast ourselves with the soothing sounds of the great maestro, counteracting the electro lullabies that annoy me from mobiles attached to adjoining cribs. Gosh these stupid dumdidums all day, repeating half-finished songs. They don't believe in verses and choruses in those plastic, battery-operated, music-replacement devices.

But, then again, these sounds blend in nicely with the cacophony of beeping machines announcing that lipids and vamins (a vitamin and mineral complex) have completed their run or that a little person's pulse is down, or their oxygen level is alarming, or they have indeed stopped breathing. So far nobody has really stopped breathing, but I keep forgetting to turn off the mattress sensor when I take Tuffel out, so the ear-drum-destroying alarm goes off three times a day (none of the babies care – it's only adult ears that fall off). But then again, we haven't wet the bed in a few days, so I'm sure that makes up for it.

So that's my life with the Tuffelmeister. Thomas asked me what I think about when I sit there with him all day. I don't really know. I just cuddle him. I go in and out of thoughts; slow my thinking activity down altogether. Watch the buses crossing Westminster Bridge. Today I counted the roof windows of County Hall. Fifteen on the lower row and eight on the top one. I thought of counting the wagons on the London Eye, but figured I can look that up online.

I just thought it could be poetic to say how many bricks there are on the wall opposite, or how many buses cross the bridge in a day. Though that's all a bit too 'trainspotty' for me. I'm busy holding my son. His hair is so soft and has a strawberry tone. Or as my hairdresser would say, a 'tint of caramel'. That's what they called it when dying my hair blonde didn't quite work out. They called it caramel. It was freaking ginger.

Nobody needs accidental ginger. Don't get me wrong, I'm the biggest fan of ginger. Just not when I tried to get Madonna-blonde. Tuffel is not Madonna blonde and he's no accidental ginger. He has a beautiful caramel honey tone to his soft fuzz, which I can't get enough of. He also still has this incredibly soft baby hair on his shoulders and back.

Softer than the softest plush. Oh, and he smells good. He smells of baby loveliness. Despite the hospital and the constant sterilising everywhere.

It's hard to believe this little bundle of loveliness has already been on morphine, pumped full of antibiotics, painkillers, and lives on space food. But if he didn't, he wouldn't be here.

And thanks to the great care of our doctors, medicine and, yes, the NHS, he is here – and that makes me very happy indeed. I'm very much in love with this little person and nothing can take that away from me.

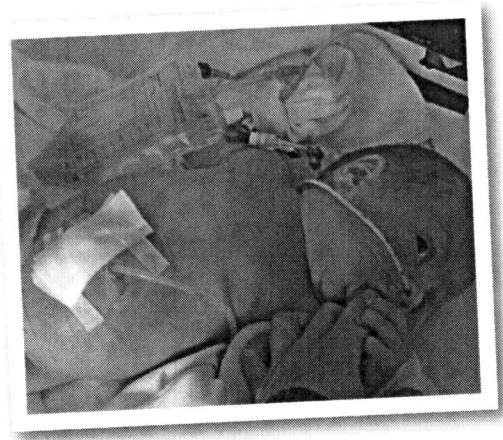

People have asked how they can help – you can help by doing something wonderful with your life. And letting me know about it. Some people have quit jobs they disliked; stopped moaning and have stepped up. "Mediocre just won't do it," I was told.

I like this a lot.

CHAPTER 3

Tuffel and the joys of motherhood

(1.5 MONTHS)

The bottles of breast milk in the freezer tell me it's the beginning of March. I have been asked not to bring in any more as the hospital freezer is almost full. At home, a list of our freezer contents would read like this: frozen seafood; spinach; fish fingers; Mum's chicken soup; my lamb stew; gel pads to soothe breast inflammation; a Migra-Cap to soothe Thomas' migraines; lactose-free ice cream; 52 bottles of breast milk; more fish fingers; the other half of the chicken that didn't fit into our pot.

I've been expressing my milk just in case one day Tuffel could have some. Diligently, every three to four hours days and night. I get up at night. I get up early in the morning. I do it in hospital looking at my baby. When I cuddle him, my breasts cry milky tears of nutritious love. When would the day come that my little boy, who can't process food, could have my milk?

It came two weeks ago!

With a cunning logistical plan, a feeding program was initiated in order to save the bits of intestines he still has. What doesn't get used, dies – so let's use what we've got!

The doctors decided to run 1ml of my milk (*my* milk!) per hour into him. It would be drained by his NJ tube that runs through his nose and sits in the top of his bowel, into a bag, along with the stomach waste. Seeing my milk bottle on top of the drip made me incredibly proud. That's my milk there, next to the selection of sterile chemical cocktails. I made that one myself! From the NJ tube bag that collects the fluids, 3ml is then re-injected into the 'red button'. The red button is actually his colon brought out of his belly (a bit like a stoma, for those who know stomas; for those who don't, a stoma is a surgically created exit point for faeces, whereas the fistula is an entry point). From there, the milk would continue its processing journey and hopefully form a poo. A poo! A real poo that would come out of his bottom – like a normal baby. Who knew we'd one day be praying for stinky nappies?

For one week, a note was left for the night nurse saying: 'If poo comes, please take a picture for mummy'. What a strange note to leave, but it was important to me. But there was no poo. It took our surgeon's little finger up his tiny bottom to release the first bit. Tuffel's facial expression during that process was priceless: his face turned bright red as if embarrassed, followed by clear vocals letting us know that this was really not on.

A few days later, we were totally convinced we smelled poo. I turned him around to smell his bottom. Nothing. But he smells! I checked the nappy. Nothing. Are we nuts? Turns out not only are we nuts, but so is he. His poo is coming out of the belly! The red button 'entry point' – nobody mentioned it might expel things too. The problem with frontal Number 2s is the increased probability of being shat upon while having a cuddle. As if my breasts didn't endure enough these days. Ah, the joys of motherhood.

Thomas and I are doing well finding a sort of routine in the strangeness of our lives. I enjoy my daily visitors and lots of quality time with the Tuffelmeister, and soothing him when the doctors and nurses have to fiddle with him. Changing the dressings of the red button, detangling the hopeless lines, solving the kinks in various ones as the alarms of the pumps go on and on.

Remember the song, *The Wheels on the Bus Go Round and Round*? For us, the lyrics are now '*The sound of the pump goes on and on! ALL day long*'.

Time to give myself a break? Given that my mum is still looking after us, I decided to leave Tuffy snoozing peacefully in her trusted arms and took an afternoon to meet up with my NCT friends – the girls with whom I learned about birthing and how to change a nappy. We shared deep insights on nipple stimulation and what baby's first stool should look like – which had been tastefully demonstrated on a doll covered in Marmite.

It was lovely to see their babies – all wireless, of course. We gathered in a beautiful house on Clapham's most popular street, eating chocolate chip cookies and talking baby talk. It was exactly how I had imagined my postnatal latte life. Except I was missing my baby. I just felt my boobs swell, cooing over five other newborns. The girls talked of sleepless nights being woken by cries. "Can you die of fatigue?" asks one new mum, her little one wearing one of these cosy baby overalls. My thoughts drift to Tuffel. He has cosy overalls, too, but try wearing clothes with tubes coming out of your belly. So we don't bother. He's as topless as mummy.

Doctors, students, nurses, parents, visitors and relatives all walk in and out of that ward. Oh well, I'll never be as young as today. But now I have a nicely veiled neighbour directly opposite me, just to make things a little more awkward.

I must be known more by my boobs than my face on that ward. I could wear a mask and they'd still know exactly who I am. I told the staff they were lucky I had my trousers on.

The other way to recognise me is by my artfully milk-stained black leather boots. Did you know that breast milk forms rather aggressive white stains? Not a situation most mothers would have to deal with – I tried water, sunflower oil, and NHS (sorry taxpayers) moisturiser to clean them. Breast milk stains are mean!

Back to the NCT group, I'm happy for everyone. I love the babies – they are soooo adorable. The girls let me cuddle them. I have a good time; I like being in a nice house, and I enjoy a clean bathroom with Molton Brown Rose and Pomegranate handwash and cream. I'm not jealous. I am not the slightest bit jealous. I love being part of Club Normal for a bit. But that night I cried. I cried big tears of self-pity, living in a small flat with nothing but Sanex Sensitive in the bathroom.

I grieved for having a baby who doesn't wake me up at night while all the normal mums get proper sleep deprivation. So to level the playing field, I got myself mastitis (inflammation of the breast with pain and fever, lumps and *ouch*!) and there was a lot of crying and very little sleeping indeed.

What snapped me out of feeling sorry for myself was the neighbouring baby in our ward: a premature sweetie whom I will always remember in his big, soft eye protectors, enjoying his phototherapy sunbed (to break down jaundice). Little Eddie (name changed for privacy) got taken away for an operation and never returned. I thought he was recovering in NICU (intensive care). Later that afternoon, I saw his mum crying and a nurse stroking her back saying, "Here is his book of health records. I know it's hard, but you still have to register his birth."

My life is good. My baby is with me, getting stronger every day. He's already over one major operation and his first two infections, and his third course of antibiotics. He's endured four attempts to fit a cannula into his foot; he's got five pumps running for him and all this at only six weeks of age. (I might rewrite the *12 Days of Christmas* with this...)

Our hospital life has its perks, too. When Tuffel cries and I get desperate, I can get help. If Sir wees all over his bed, someone else comes to change the sheets. If he spits his dummy out, someone else will sterilise it. A nurse will wipe his poo for me. Hospital is social. I am never on my own. Chats on tap and tea on the house. If I'm not sure if something's okay, I can call a doctor. (S)he is usually in the room.

Of course, given the choice, I'd go for the hardship of 'normal' motherhood any day. I don't have that choice so I might as well adapt and really enjoy what I do have. *That* is the teaching of Tuffel.

Tuffmeister is being discussed by many experts as he's such a rare case. What's next? After being advised that a transplant really is the last resort, our latest meeting with our specialist team, led by gastroenterologist Jonathan Hind, went the opposite direction: a transplant now sounds like a great option for him. "Let's get him assessed and make a plan to vaccinate him to get on the list sooner rather than later," they say.

We want his liver to be healthy, so we'll only need one organ. The problem is, living on TPN long-term increases the chances of the liver giving in, meaning a transplant of two organs would be necessary. Small bowel transplants are a relatively new thing – in London, at the time of writing this, only eight kids have had one thus far. I've met one of them. A lovely five year old. And yes, she's doing well, but life with a donor organ means a lifelong intake of immunosuppressive drugs. When you or I lie in bed with a cold, it's in the comfort of our own home; a transplant patient would be in hospital. It's a big deal. I'm not going to talk about the side effects of the drugs – I only know they are harsh. I don't yet want to know…

But what does sound exciting is the possibility of Tuffel eating real food and the possibility of a wireless life.

Three days ago another miracle occurred. A dream came true. An experience so blissfully wonderful and longed for I could Tweet it until the end of time. Alright, I won't Tweet it that long. I might not Tweet it at all. But I will share it with you. I was finally allowed to take him to my breast. He could have my milk. After five weeks of sucking dummies and little fingers, he'd finally be getting the real deal! After each breastfeeding session the doctors will do to him what they would for many other hard-partying Brits on a Saturday night: pump out his stomach. Luckily, he's already wired up for that.

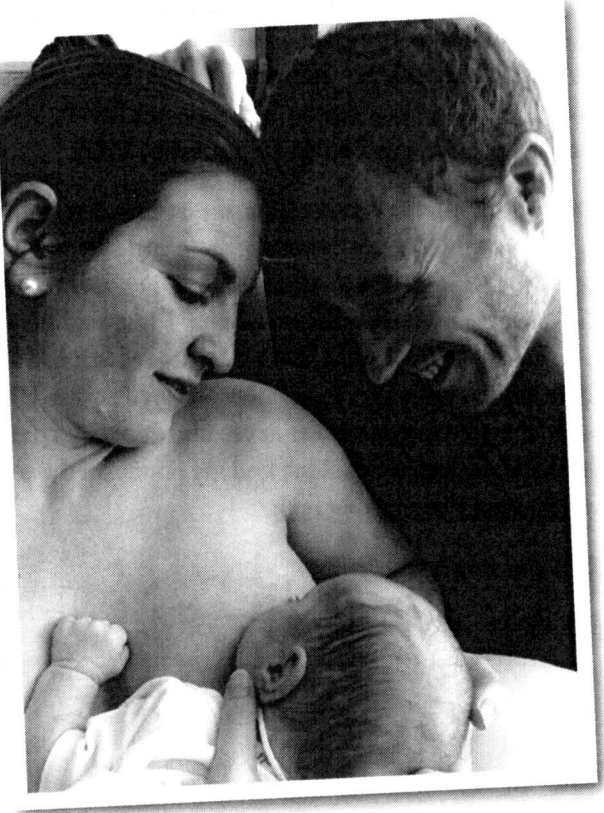

So when he latched on and started sucking, imagine his surprise at the sweet liquid coming out… his pupils enlarged. Mine must have too as we tripped on our first milk-induced oxytocin high together. Ah, the joy of motherhood! I cried. It was so beautiful; it felt so right. The feeling was incredible, and to see him loving it too was glorious. And afterwards he fell into his first milk coma, tired and satisfied, and I've never felt more emotionally fulfilled. I never knew you could love so much.

His adorability is rising on a daily basis. I'm crazy about his facial expressions. Admittedly, the baby smell is compromised a little due to his colon confusion, but he more than makes up for that by just being Tuffel.

I am as baby-brained as they come – at least I've got that in common with Club Normal. The other day, my mum called me to ask when a visitor was coming, and to check the calendar I searched for my phone. I just couldn't find it anywhere on the couch, though I was so sure it had been there just a minute ago. I got rather annoyed at this. Here I am making a conscious effort not to lose things and then… I realised the reason I couldn't find my phone on the couch was because I was talking on it.

Will you sing it with me?

'Ah, the joys of motherhood!'

CHAPTER 4

Life is sweet. Sometimes.

(2.5 MONTHS)

This living miracle who is our baby is giving us a new sense of purpose, vitality and appreciation every day. I have mutated into the mum who tells everyone how gorgeous her son is, while shoving an endless series of photos in your face. "Look at him, isn't he gorgeous? And here! And *here*! And this one." (All photos being pretty much the same, except for eyes opening and closing.) Please don't ever do this to me.

But you see, my baby is particularly gorgeous. "Look at him, now he moved his mouth! Oh look! He wrinkled his forehead – he's so cute when he wrinkles his forehead." Friends are those people who enthusiastically follow my cooing with a "Yes! He is ever so cute," ignoring the tubes and wires that would probably distract anyone who wasn't used to it into all sorts of worried thinking. If you can't beat her, join her, they think, and echo my delight. "Oh there – he pursed his lips. Such cute little lips. And his eyes – gee, look at his eyes. Let's take another picture." Meanwhile, he'll pull a face, going cross-eyed, presenting his double chin and triple neck. Okay, that photo I'll delete. And the one where he sleeps on me with mouth open, the tube splitting his cheek in two chubby halves and dribble running out, I'll keep that to myself too.

Hospital life is far from dull. The idea that I'd turn in my glamorous life for one of endless nappy changing and leaking breasts while my work desk collects dust has faded into the mist of my many unlived futures. The future is a funny thing, because it doesn't exist yet – and when it does, it immediately loses its status of being the future. And, if we consider the future as a cluster of possibilities, then to worry about the future would subsequently involve the question: which one? One would have to pick another possible future that looks less worry-worthy. (Yes that was the Tip of the Day, very subtly hidden).

I'm not saying this flippantly. I have plenty of opportunities to worry about the future. Every parent in the Neonatal Unit worries about the future of their baby. You can divide the members of our exclusive club into two groups: those who lose themselves worrying about the future, and those who use the day to collect the nectar of love from the ephemeral flower that is their child. Group One looks worn out. Their visiting sessions decline rapidly, as it's all 'too much'. Extreme cases in Group One don't even make it through the door. Group Two is still smiling.

In our unit – the HDU (or High Dependency Unit) – it's transient; the babies change almost every day, certainly every week. But I've found myself in a nice little group of long-timers with two other mums after we got chatting to each other. The others both have premature babies who, at three months of age, are still younger than Tuffel, who is now two months old. Except they are, of course, one month ahead. WTF? Born at 26 weeks, even after 12 weeks these babies are only now approaching their due dates and are almost the size of a newborn. Most babies in the ward are early birds. One of these preemies is still on breathing support and keeps falling asleep at her mummy's breast when she tries to feed.

The other one had a bowel operation and has a heart condition. I found out the doctors suggested to his mum that she let him go and allow them to turn off the ventilator because the brain and lung bleeding was too serious to give the baby a good chance in life. He'd be too damaged, they said. This mum made a very brave decision. She said NO. She had faith in her baby. Are you ready to hear about another miracle? The bleeding subsided; there was no damage to the brain after all; the heart condition turned out to be very, very mild and the bowel could be operated upon. They are ready to go home next month. I am thrilled for them. That kind of story sends chills up and down my spine.

Then we have the Muslim couple I mentioned earlier, challenging my topless routine with the mere presence of veils. I have an ingrained respect for other cultures and religions, so I did feel awkward taking my clothes off in front of them and their extended family. But then again, I have to live according to my own values and skin-to-skin care is the best I can do for the emotional development of my child and our mutual wellbeing. I might have mentioned how much I love feeling him close to me. If I haven't mentioned it 100 times yet, I shall be approaching it by the end of this chapter.

I noticed the note on Mustafa's cot (his name has been changed for privacy) requesting that blood should not be taken from his right foot. I pondered what kind of religious tradition wouldn't allow blood being taken from the right foot. I am aware some cultures refuse blood transfusions, so it must have been something in that vein (are you liking the pun?). Or maybe the little one had been blessed in a ceremony and the sacred foot therefore mustn't be touched.

Every Tuesday is parents' group, where we enjoy M&S chocolates (get jealous now). I avoided parents' group for the first month or so because it just seemed too much to eat cookies and talk about our problems. And I was often caught up in cuddling time or a medical procedure. I also find that it's easy to emphasize one's difficulties in a group situation, which leads me down the path of feeling sorry for myself, and I value my positive state of mind.

There are two ways to deal with challenges. One is to retreat inside oneself: I isolate myself in my own thoughts and keep myself to myself. It feels justified and as if I need to sort it out myself anyway. The other way is to reach out and connect. It doesn't make the actual situation better, but it lightens the burden created by personal thinking. By 'personal thinking', I mean all those little thoughts running around that clog up the peaceful feeling that's present when my mind is quiet. Having said all this, once I started going to parents' group, it became my sacred activity. Connecting with others, sharing our stories and looking at our experiences from different viewpoints proved extremely valuable. A good cuppa and a chat really does go a long way.

And last Tuesday, my veiled neighbour and her husband were there too – it turned out they are super nice and very approachable. So I just asked what was up with this note about the blood. Turns out, Mustafa had a blood clot and got some medicine for it, so therefore the right leg shouldn't be used for taking blood. There went my religious fantasies.

Mustafa is a super-cute baby. He reminds me of Eddie.

Then we got another neighbour baby in HDU: Casper, a little early bird with an accumulation of health challenges from not being able to breathe due to a misshaped windpipe, cleft palate, and what-have-you. His mum, Claire, is an editor and a writer and works in design; his dad, Tom, is a journalist. They are lovely, warm-hearted, spirited people with an extensive vocabulary: a combination I highly appreciate. I'd always meet Claire in the milk expressing room, and we'd have similar timings coming to the hospital. If you think Tuffel's story is challenging, Casper's journey is nowhere less dramatic. Not that this is a competition. Casper keeps our adrenaline running high as his vital stats are a rollercoaster ride and I've witnessed his oxygen saturation drop from 90% to 7% with the red lights going off several times a day. The colour of Claire's face would dip alongside Casper's oxygen levels. Mine too, because I'd be holding my breath for them.

The joy of having them in the room was short-lived, though – they had to go back to Intensive Care. The route you want to take is from right to left up the hallway. Usually they start in the Neonatal Intensive Care Unit (NICU), go next door to High Dependency (HDU), followed by the Special Care Baby Unit (SCBU), then home! But unfortunately, there is a lot of zigzagging along the way. It's a bit like Monopoly here. Do Not Pass Go, Do Not Collect £200.

But not everyone goes back on track. Sure, the move from High Dependency back to Intensive Care isn't pleasant, but at least it's a horizontal move. My very cute new Muslim friend – whom, after the ice-breaking parent group, I would visit daily – was taken for an operation. I assumed he was in Intensive Care to recover, after all that's how it usually works, but I hadn't seen his parents in a while. I then learned why: vertical move. Unexpectedly, he had more than one heart problem and couldn't make it, even on a bypass… you can feel the heavy atmosphere after a loss. The gratitude I feel in my heart for Tuffel mixes with the weight of the sad realities around us. Is this just some sort of Russian roulette?

The fact that many more babies get saved than die, remains. And yet the shock of losing those you get to know is harsh. Tears speak deeper than words.

Every now and then, babies who've made it home come to visit and the joy and uproar is always beautiful to see: the nurses rush out to say hello, eyes shining bright, with big smiles and cries of "Haven't you grown! Look at you – you look amazing!". It must be so rewarding to see the fruit of your labour. The number of thankyou cards decorating the walls speak for themselves. I look at them with hope. I want to join the ranks of happy families sending in a card with a massive "Thank you for all your help – we are so happy, the three of us."

For now, Tuffy is doing amazingly. Looking at it, he has a high quality of life: daily cuddles skin to skin, and three breastfeeding sessions. Undivided attention. No phone interrupts us – all mobiles must be on silent – and I have no

Life is sweet. Sometimes.

chores to attend to. No washing machines, food shopping, cleaning, appointments, no rush. Okay, there are doctors and nurses who fiddle and observe stats and change fluids and lines. There are vampire nurses sucking his blood; the number of prick wounds he has on his hands and especially feet I am learning to ignore. He gets stung at least twice a day for blood sugar levels, and twice a week, they take several tubes of his life juice to amend his nutrition and check for infection levels. Now, he hardly flinches when he gets pricked. Let's say that besides all he has to endure, he has a wonderful life. And what he has to endure, he is taking like a man. Though most men would moan more. He takes it like a Tuffel. He certainly deserves his Viking hat.

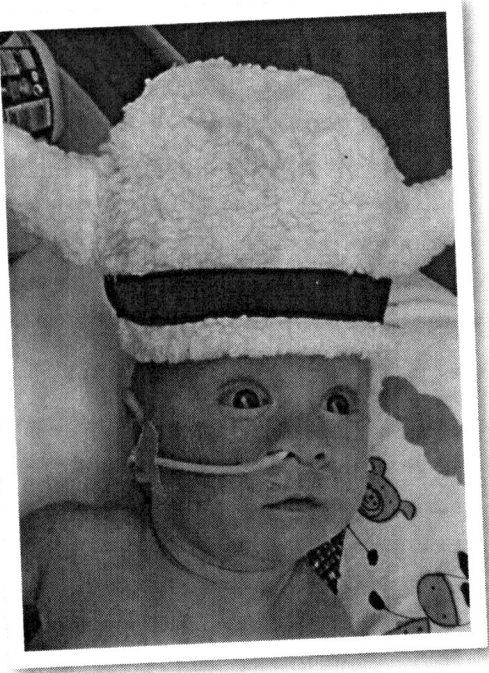

I can report big improvements on the poo front as well. No more frontal poos. After a week of daily rectal washouts, Mr Tuffel is shitting like we would after a spicy Indian meal. I'm aware that's not good language, but it's great news. It would be rude to withhold it. We must celebrate the advancements. Today Thomas did his first poo-nappy change. I marked it in the calendar. I tried to hide a look of self-satisfaction. I failed.

We are learning about a possible transplant and what that would all mean. The first year would be spent in and out of hospital for tests and whatnots. He would have a stoma for six to 18 months to check for potential rejection. A stoma involves a bag collecting his outputs (a rather literal bowel opening). After six to 18 months there would be another big operation connecting the ends of the new bowel. He would need about 15 drugs twice a day. The immunosuppressive drug has to be administered with gloves and apron on while wearing a mask. How will I explain this to my child? "Honey eat this, you need that, but mummy mustn't even breathe while it's out. Daddy just had to go upstairs with your little sister so they don't get ill, but seriously, it's good for you."

The side effects are manageable. The word 'managing' is shifting meaning for me: it's no longer about juggling tasks or delegating, but has become much more about 'coping' and 'life-death balance through necessary drug intake'. Side effects need to be closely monitored. They rank from not feeling so good to blood cancer. No wonder I didn't want to hear too much about it.

Let's talk about some lighter things. As you'll be thrilled to hear, my milk production continues apace. I am a serious contender for the Lactation Award of 2012 – in an attempt to do something great I marched up to the nurse in charge of the Neonatal Unit's milk bank (which stores pasteurised breast milk for newborns whose mums can't breastfeed them) and asked blatantly: "What has been your biggest donation of milk to date?" She smiled at me. "Why would you like to know that?" " Because I want to beat it!" I like a crazy challenge and focusing my energy on something positive in all this madness can only be good. The response had my face turn as white as milk: 50 litres.

Shit. Moo! But I'd already said it, hadn't I? Now I'd better start squeezing. It's official: my goal is to become the biggest milk donor in the hospital's history.

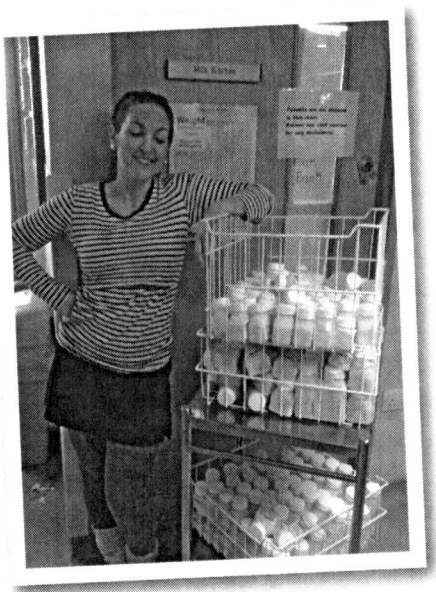

In this picture (previous page) you see 20 litres of my produce. Please don't tell me about the London shop that made ice cream from breast milk – you'd be number 52. It was called Baby Gaga. Lady Gaga sued them for misusing her brand. Plus, what were they thinking? Who wants ice cream made from a stranger's breast milk? My milk is for babies who NEED it. It's not so easy for mums to achieve good milk production when they get distressed, or if the baby arrives too early. So quite a few preemies lack the most important substance for their growth. Milk production is mental. Just like me.

I'm expressing every four hours or so, regardless of Tuffel having his faux feed. I'm expressing no matter where I am. Here's how this works: your boobs fill up to bursting limits regardless of whether you have the pump ready or not. So have your pump ready. Baby-brain forgetfulness and this necessity aren't a good combination. Nature didn't think that one through. That's why Thomas now knows how to assemble a breast pump and find the bits and pieces from two models in the steriliser. That's what I call an achievement.

I'm happy to report that the cup holder in Leicester Square cinema does fit my hand-held pump perfectly. And if you saw the *Muppets* on the 6th of March and heard a rhythmic squeaky noise in the middle of the film, now you know what it was. It was surreal to go to the movies. Walking to the bus stop from central London at night, I wondered which part was the dream. We looked like a normal family. Thomas and me celebrating my mum's birthday with the Muppet movie, having a laugh. You wouldn't know what we've been through; that we have a two-month old in Intensive Care. On the bright side, we didn't have to organise a babysitter.

Another dream came true: for the first time, we were allowed to leave the Unit. With Tuffel! I had been wondering when my cable-baby would feel fresh air on his skin. Would it be six months? A year? When we got out of hospital? There is a world out there I'd love to show him. There are birds singing and flowers blooming and the sun shining… The doctors talked about the possibility of taking him off TPN for an hour soon, so I gathered that by summer I could take him for a stroll. Maybe finally introduce him to Thomas' nieces, Scarlet and Daisy. The girls are nine and seven now and really want to meet their cousin.

It turns out that asking the same questions of different people yields amazing results. One consultant makes it sound as if it could be months until I can take him out. He tells me how complicated and unlikely it is to happen anytime soon. He 'manages expectations'. My mind is geared for power not for restriction. So I am reacting to his comments with irritation driven to prove him wrong.

He says things like "I don't want to give you false hopes" as if there was such a thing as false hope. Hope is a concept beyond 'true' or 'false'. Or "We are looking at a very different person from the one we met two months ago," while going over Tuffel's wonderfully stable charts. What a funny thing to say. No, we're not. We are looking at Tuffel. His potential unfolding. That was him all along. I can see that because I don't look at problems as much as I focus on possibilities. But then again I don't get sued (or threatened of this) when things go the other way. Some doctors at very protective and understandably so. But others are rooted in possibility thinking. And they are the ones who change the world.

It was just after Mother's Day when we had this conversation: "When Tuffel's stable on dextrose, he'll go on saline and when he's stable on that then maybe you can try and take him out a little." The next day he went on dextrose. Dr. Hammad Khan was in charge – he's a lovely, soft-spoken, smart and open consultant. The kind who will kneel because you're on the floor so as to not tower over you. Plus, a team of open-minded nurses was on shift. To my delight, the answer to "when would I be able to take Tuffel out?" therefore changed from "one day at some point maybe" to "now". Tuffel found himself lifted into an old-fashioned tank of a buggy, enjoying the blue walls outside his own corner of Room 2. I even showed him the water cooler – how exciting, the 50 shades of blue.

Okay, time for more drama now.

Tuffel's tummy tube fell out. It shouldn't be possible because it's held by a balloon on the other end (inside his stomach). But it happened nevertheless and when I discovered it, the uproar was big. Nurses, doctors, surgeons trying to stick it back in. It was too late. The hole had closed. I tried saying "open sesame" three times but even that let us down.

He now looks like he has two belly buttons. Shame about the modelling career, I know. Opposite is a diagram of the Tuffmeister I made to give you an idea of how it all works.

This could have been quite a problem, with all the milk bloating up his inside. Because it had nowhere to go, it could have come back up and aspirated into the lungs which doctors are always worried about. But what I really like about my boy is how gracefully he jumps such hurdles. All the milk came out by the one tube he had left, and he didn't throw up or show any signs of discomfort. He got a new tube into his tummy through his nose.

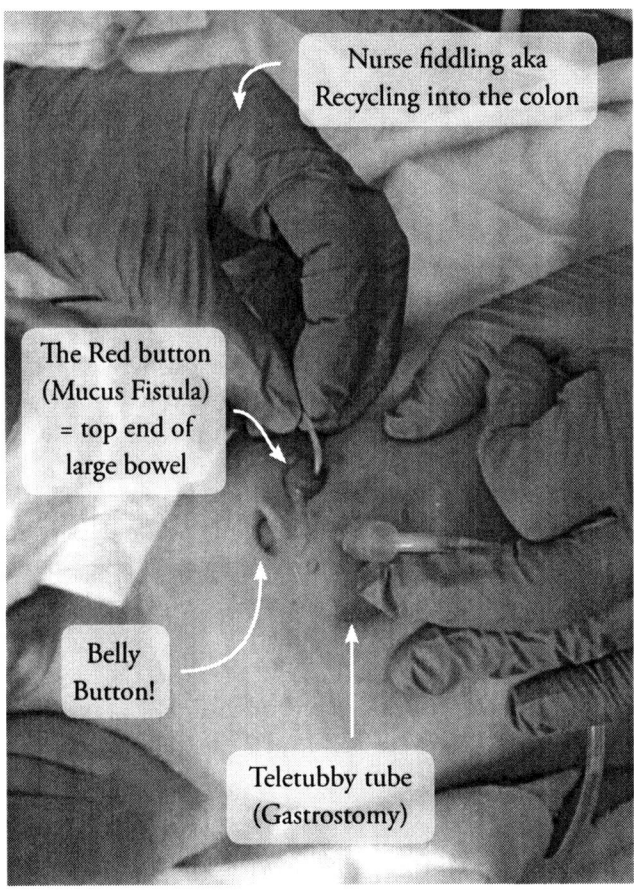

In some ways, things are very similar to 'normal' motherhood. I multitask like crazy. But instead of cooking and changing my baby at the same time, I've got the Rottweiler milk-expressing machine on my right nipple while I soothe Tuffy with my index finger (left hand) and open up syringe packaging with the other hand while defending *his* hand from the Vampire Nurses. Again. Prick the heel, but leave his hand alone, I beg you. We've had this before. I know it's procedure. But didn't you want a result? There is no blood in the hand.

Vaccinations were carried out and we can't even be bothered to make too big a deal out of it. Needles in my baby? Sure, why not. Where would you like to put them this time? Why not try a leg today? He's got two. Okay, take both legs. Five vaccines in one go? Is that all you got? At least take his bloods today as well. And they do.

He cries for a little and then he's busy sucking my finger again. We don't have much time for staying upset. There are cuddles to be enjoyed in between all this medical madness.

When I was little it took four adults to pin me down and give me one shot. So I thought Tuffel should hold my hand while I got my bloods taken to qualify as an official milk donor. He did. And I didn't feel a thing.

CHAPTER 5

The art of empowerment or how to save a baby from the operating table

(Tuffel is now 3 months old)

How can you thrive in a world of uncertainty? With so many variables in the way, how can we make the right decisions? When things are overwhelming, isn't it easier to sit back and hope for the best? I have a son in hospital and his fate is decided by the gods in white. Who nowadays wear green. Or Prada (depending on the type of god). My decision-making as a mother is compromised. When every nappy change, every millilitre of milk, every bowel movement is monitored and charted, where is the power that one expects from carrying responsibility?

I had a dream the first week after Tuffel was born: I was inside a ghost ride 3D movie. I was walking or riding along and monsters jumped at me out of the dark night sky. There were torturing murderers trying to get me and I ran for my life again and again. I tried to get out of this movie but I couldn't. I was stuck inside this alternate reality of the horror script and it became rather real in that context. There was no end in sight. I just had to sit back and endure the ride. The dream was a pretty direct translation of my situation, of course. Not getting out of the real-life nightmare, trapped in uncertainty and impending pain and doom. It is so mean when someone you love deeper than you thought possible should be taken away from you in the cruellest fashion. It's a really painful scenario.

Have you ever 'woken up' in your dream and taken control? Realised whilst sleeping that you're dreaming and therefore you can do anything? I feel a shift in my consciousness; an elevation and expansion in my mind when I wake up in my dream. I then do things I couldn't do in my daytime body – from deep-sea diving without the need of oxygen, to running at the speed of light, or calling on spiritual teachers for an advanced soul lesson and, most of all, flying. I love flying.

I also start making up the story. Or change the course of one. What a fun thing to do at night.

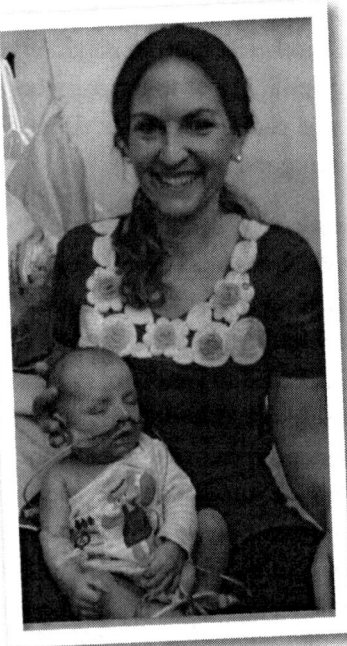

But what's even more powerful is to 'wake up' in life and realise it's you who creates the story. Even in the most dire circumstances, when we think we may not have any control of our circumstances, we can wake up and take some control.

Here is Tuffel practising elevating his consciousness.

Because of the missing gastrostomy (the surgical opening that had closed when his tummy tube fell out), the surgeons were keen to replace it at their earliest convenience. A tube inserted through his nose and throat into the stomach acted as a temporary replacement, and while nobody likes having a tube in each nostril, interestingly, it works better than the direct plumbing we had before. So, we requested that it stay. And that the doctors don't operate. While other parents decide on how many layers of babygrows they should wrap their junior in, we get to choose between tubes in nostril versus hole in stomach. All better than a hole in the head.

The two-tube scenario makes sense to me, even from a fashion perspective. His poor nostrils are shaping nicely like a dragon – so might as well not have a lopsided dragon nose. Discussions followed, though not about the visual aspects of the dragon-nose effect as surgeons are oblivious to aesthetics. Our surgeon agreed to speak to the specialist and ask for his opinion, too. The next day, Thomas got the news: we are operating on Monday. We don't need to speak to the specialist.

Nightmare! No! That's not what we wanted. Why? It's safer and better, we are told. End of story. What could we do? Say NO! We can say NO. So we did. "So you are refusing treatment?" Thomas was very polite but firm. "No, we want a proper meeting and discussions to hear what changed and take it from there."

To cut a long story short, all the other doctors agreed with us, including our specialist, Dr. Hind, whom I refer to as "da man". It's amusing to see the relationship between the medics. Dr. Hind trained under many of the Neonatal team and they look upon him with some sort of parental fondness. But he's now a specialist and knows so much more than them in the area of our concern. When they spend days debating how to increase this or that input, driving us crazy with being too conservative in approach, he's the one pushing for more, because we can and we must always try to push the boundaries in a controlled manner. He's not just Jonathan who was trained here. He da man who knows now. He da man!

There is absolutely no need to operate. Had we not stood our ground, Tuffel would have been under the knife. Just like that.

Understandably, the hospital environment can seem overwhelming. We woke up to our power. And changed the fate of our son.

Since Tuffel did so well on his little trip, our time out of the ward has been extended to one hour a day. In that hour, he is disconnected from his feed and connected to saline to keep hydrated and keep the line open. We now have permission to leave the building and pace merrily around the hospital square with the water feature outside, waving at Big Ben till we are dizzy. The other day, a nurse sent us off without attaching the pump he needs. "Excuse me, he needs to be on the saline pump," I said. "No, no," she responded, "you can go ahead." She was a very experienced nurse – a sister. You can't get any higher than that. She had been working there for so long, her name had faded off her name tag. She knows what she's doing.

But I know that to keep a long line running (that's the line through which he gets all his nutrition), something has to go through it at all times to keep it open. So you can't just disconnect it. According to her, you can!

I had two voices in my head. One said: "Listen and learn, she knows better than you. Don't piss her off – she's looking after your son!" The other one said: "You know what you need; stick with that and learn if needed later." I put my foot down and got my pump. Had I not done this, his line would have been destroyed. To put another one in, you have to find a vein and get a tiny line to run all the way close to the heart. It takes between one hour and two days of trying and it's not nice for the little one. Our neighbouring baby in the Unit lost a considerable amount of weight in the time it took them to fix hers. To plump up babies is not an easy task and every gram counts. Our little neighbour had not been showing good access to her veins so her line was run through her head!

A few minutes later, blood was in the line. I alerted the nurse. She didn't seem too concerned as she increased a pressure and turned to do other things again. The blood remained in the line and as time was ticking, I got more and more tense in my stomach. When the blood clots, the line will be blocked and stops working. That means a new line is needed – was today just the end of the line? There was nothing I could do but watch. I'd already annoyed her with my demands. How far would I push things?

What if I found out later that the line had blocked? I would say: "I tried to get her attention and she didn't listen to me." That's victim perspective justifying itself. But I know about waking up in the dream. I know about taking charge. So I left the room and asked for a doctor. I interrupted them talking, even though that's rude – I learned that as a kid. It's weird how I still feel a bit like a kid interrupting the grownups when doctors are convening. Wait till you're spoken to! Lucky I'm rude, so I just burst in and asked: "Am I paranoid, or is blood in the line a bit of a problem?"

"Well, how long has it been there?"

"Ten minutes or so." The doctor dropped everything to sort this out.

They had told us that surviving hospital is a great challenge and I am beginning to see why. Even though the care is generally outstanding, people make mistakes. Admittedly, Tuffel's care plan is out of the ordinary. And his nurses change every second day. It is confusing what he needs. It's just not how it's usually done.

So I brainstormed a solution with a senior nurse – one who believes in better – and she drew up a plan that outlines it all clearly. I then asked her to also produce a schedule and attach it to the front of his folder. Done. It's quite fun to see the consultants and surgeons referring to this plan as if it were The Bible. It's written down, so it's official. I just smile when they quote it back to me.

I feel amazing. Empowered. I created a clarity for my baby and I am hands-on involved in his care. By now I understand the chart, and, dare I say it, I know all the numbers by heart. I even do the complex recycling process into his colon with syringes, tubes and stoma bags.

Finally I don't have to wait and despair if a nurse is not on time. If acidic stomach juices are leaking through the bag, I don't have to worry about the damage to his skin. I know how to remove a stoma bag, and plaster on a new one. They should employ crying babies at schools – when a baby cries, you learn really fast.

A month ago this would have been impossible. It just proves we can learn about anything. If even I can learn stoma care, you can get a grip on your situation – however challenging that may be. But I dare a rocket scientist to understand Tuffel-care.

And I dare you to do something you think is impossible. It feels incredible.

The cool thing is that I didn't have to think big or step up or motivate myself. I don't need to overcome anything or fight any demons. All I did was listen to my intuition. Listen to the obvious. And follow it. Everyone has that connection to their own wisdom; it's merely a question of slowing down enough to hear it. Miracles need that quiet space to unfold (and be noticed).

There is a lot to be said for the spiritual care Tuffel has been receiving from all the thoughts and prayers directed his way. Not all babies unfold that effortlessly. There are a lot of ups and downs in the ward – alarms sounding and dramas occurring. Stressed doctors and nurses running around from emergency to emergency.

Tuffy is continuing to thrive and I can't be grateful enough for that. And as he's done so well with his blood sugar levels, we now have two hours to stroll around. Soon my NCT friends will come and we'll be yummy mummies at the AMT cafe in the hospital lobby and whip our breasts out whilst sipping cappuccinos and eating our single slices of cellophane-wrapped carrot cake. (NCT stands for national childcare trust and first time mummies meet through birth preparation classes and connect to share their adventure of being a new mummy).

It's Easter, and as a breast feeder I've got the best excuse in the world to eat chocolate! But alas, my lactose-intolerant digestively challenged sweetheart failed to satisfy my sweet tooth. Thank God for the Easter Bunny! I might not believe in Santa anymore, but I've seen the Easter Bunny! The real Easter Bunny rides a Harley Davidson and wears black leather, did you know? I didn't, until he appeared in the Neonatal Ward distributing chocolate eggs (and yes, the Harley-Davidson Riders Club really does come round every Easter to give out chocolates).

And Tuffel also had his first ever bath! Call it spring cleaning. His lines have to stay out of the water – the blue glove in the picture is the nurse making sure that happens – and his bags are flying around in their multiple colours. It's very Eastery indeed. Tuffy loved it.

Look at our faces here – proud as can be having won the 'who keeps their babies out of the water the longest competition'. Ten weeks! Don't try that at home.

Soon we'll be going to King's College Hospital to get all his transplant assessments done – the tests to see whether he is actually suitable for a transplant. Fingers crossed and hearts open it will all be dandy!

The art of empowerment

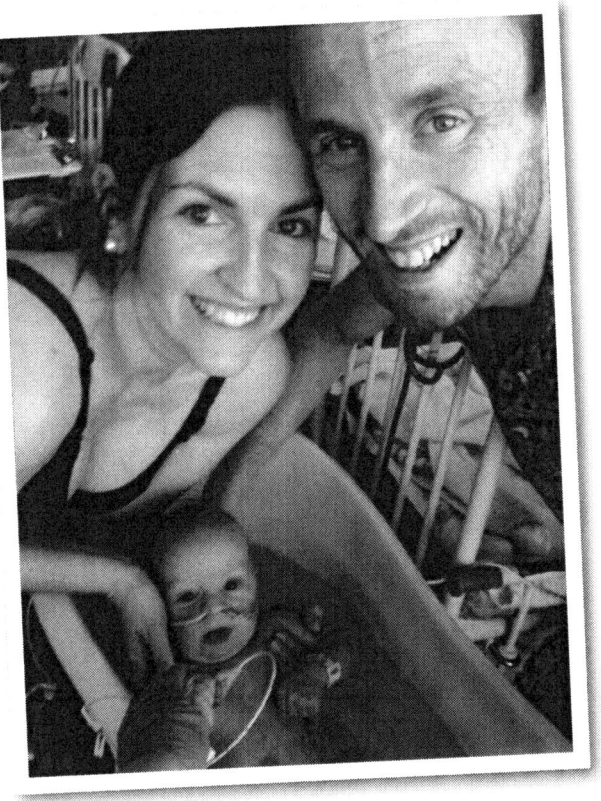

CHAPTER 6

Prince Tuffel at King's Hospital from surviving to thriving

(4 MONTHS)

Ding ding goes my phone to alert me of a text message. In a minute it will ding again. I am one of those people compelled to find out who dinged me immediately. I have to find out before it ding dings again. Nobody needs the reminder ding. That's annoying. But today ding ding is music to my ears. I will happily listen to it again. I will not move.

I had been crying non-stop after being abandoned in a hospital cubicle, left to my own devices. I didn't even have all the supplies I needed to get on with Tuffel's nursing care. I didn't have all the nerves I needed, either. We'd been transferred to King's College Hospital for a few days in order to get all the transplant assessments done in one fell swoop, and it was meant to be an amazing, fun experience. That's how I had envisioned it. We would relax and spend the night together, being cosy and enjoying each other's company, the Tuffmeister and me.

Three tearful breakdowns later, I realised I had no idea what taking a baby out of their known environment could do. He was beside himself. I speak three languages pretty fluently, a fourth sufficiently, but I can't understand what my baby is saying. Or I can't do anything about it – or both. All I hear is "Raaaaawww raaaaaww! Aaaargh! Cough cough naaaa. Eaaaah WaaaaaaAAAA!" Repeat/ad lib.

Let me guess: you are a) hungry; b) tired; c) you don't like my dress. You want to a) maul my nipples; b) cuddle; c) shoot the nurse; d) all of the above. I'm glad he's not going to write a customer feedback form rating his experience because nobody wants a one-star review.

So here is a 12-week-old boy who has lived in a 26-degrees Celsius intensive care unit for all his little life. Mummy is the person who cuddles, sings and launches kissing attacks all the time. She appears way too late in the day and leaves in the evening. Daddy is the guy with hair on his face who pulls funny faces and looks a lot at his rectangle with lights (oh, we like lights too and one day will take over Daddy's iPhone). The people in purple uniforms probe him and sometimes cuddle, and he knows beeping of machines, his little cot, the blue walls of the ward.

And now here he is in a big boy's bed in a white room that's quiet. No beeping. With air con. No-one wears purple and Mummy just won't go away. That part is the easiest to handle (I suppose). But even saying that comes out as "WAAAAAA!" I had asked if I should bring all my nursing gear. Not the sexy outfit, I mean the actual syringes, enteral drainage bags and tubes. Plus nappies and wipes and the cot mobile.

I was told that King's Hospital would have nursing supplies and given that the title of hospital points to it being a major health institution, I accepted that I wasn't actually travelling to a Third World country. Turns out I should have trusted my instincts (and taken a sexy nursing outfit). Each hospital uses different types of syringes. So the ones they have here are cheaper (I am told), which I don't mind so much, but they won't hook to my tubes. This I do mind and I need adapters. Which were brought from some stock room but are such fiddly annoying things that tend to fall off in the middle of aspirating gastric fluids (not so pleasant). In other words, I get yellow half-digested liquid that doesn't come out in the wash, all over myself. It should colour coordinate with the breast milk stains, at least!

And it turned out they also didn't have the stoma bags we use, they didn't have the drainage bags, they didn't have the feeding tube. So now what? I end up using mine for longer and sterilising them. At St. Thomas' we throw things away. Here we reuse. (Having grown up in a green household in Germany, I got quite fond of the sterilising and reusing.) It took eight hours to get all the stuff together and sorted out. In the meantime, I was left on my own in the cubicle and had to get on with things. I am used to having two or three nurses in the room and access to people and resources at all times. Suddenly I fnd myself completely isolated and forlorn.

This picture shows Tuffy ever so securely fastened in his stretcher for the transfer. I noted that it is called a Pegasus and asked if it could fly. The driver reassured me: "Only out of the back of the car". But what do you do if you are of bigger proportions than the Pegasus would allow to carry? Well, then they will arrange for a Megasus. Which apparently has the logo of a rhino.)

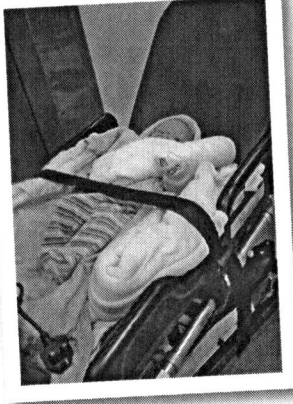

Kicking and screaming, I was. And so was he – gosh I couldn't tell who did what anymore. Dirty bags and cables just everyfreakingwhere. It was Sunday so hardly anyone was around and the nurse in charge was busy. I didn't buzz her because I didn't know what to buzz for. Nobody knows what to do better than me; you can see every new care person getting completely confused when Tuffel's situation is explained to them. When they say "he's unique" what they really mean is "I haven't got a clue what to do with him".

Plus, I don't have time to wait for people. He needs care now. By 6:30pm I was finished. My nurse comes in: "Are you okay?" No I'm not. You would think the tears streaming down my cheeks would give her a clue. "Well, let me know if there is anything I can do to help you." I don't know what someone who is clearly too busy to come in at the times she needs to can really do for me.

At 8:30pm I started shivering. My milk ducts blocked up and my breasts started to hurt. Not another onset of mastitis please, nooooo! I felt feverish. I was cold. The aircon was blowing heat. I had pulled a muscle in my back the night before, so every move was painful on top of it all. My eyes were burning. So that's my wonderful experience of spending time with my baby. Would the night be okay?

In Germany we have an expression that you 'walk on your gums', referring to one's last reserve of nerves and energy, the teeth having worn down. I was crawling on my gums. I begged the night nurse to take over Tuffel's care. It is her job, after all. She just said, "But of course!" and smiled. She was brilliant and kind. I couldn't really sleep on the plastic mattress, but I could lie back and think of England. That didn't really work (and neither did thinking of Germany) so I tried calming my thoughts. Even if thoughts don't always calm that way, I did tire of it and that was the goal in the first place.

To my absolute delight and surprise, Tuffel is a great sleeper and super peaceful at night. At 6am I took him out of his cot for a breastfeed and cuddle. I don't know why I had tried feeding sitting on the bed and on the hard-backed chair. If my back had a voice, its prolonged screaming would have given me tinnitus. Lying down is so much cosier. So there we were, lying, enjoying booby bliss. Finally comfortable. And then we both fell asleep. It was so harmonious, so simple, so long awaited.

Moments of normality are precious to us. Finally, to lie in a bed with my son for the first time – after 90 days – tears of joy yet again. When he came back the next day, Thomas said he felt like a real family for the first time in that little room. It gave us the privacy every young family needs to get to know itself as a new entity. So in that white cubicle of 3x3m, we finally had some space.

The tests went well. One of the blood tests sounded like hell – Thomas tried to defend the hand, which was dry as usual. I chose to talk to a medical student who wanted to learn about the case. We were so busy. People meeting with us non-stop, coming to our little abode, but I had Tuffel on me or next to me so I didn't mind at all.

So far, all looks normal. Then one consultant broke the news that the liver tests showed levels of inflammation, so we should take some tissue from the liver to see how long we've got till that one packs up. It's the kind of information we don't want. But Dr. Hind, our specialist, disagreed and said it was all normal in the ultrasound, so no worries. Yet.

The feeding specialist said that of the surgical babies, he was the best feeder she'd ever seen. After that horrid day one, Tuffel was peaceful and gorgeous. I didn't really want to go back to the 1.27 square metres at our local hospital (St Thomas'), but I did miss my people there. Being away made me realise what I have there and also what I don't. We need to fight for more space. He's a big boy and he shouldn't stay stuck in a neonatal unit. I will certainly let go of my silly angst about having the most shouty baby in the room. My son is a lion (toothless, thank God) in a field of kittens. Premature babies really do sound like kittens when they cry. Tuffel has a roar. His middle name Leo is certainly appropriate.

All in all we won't know much more until all the doctors from their respective fields have met and debated what the best way forward is. Whether to transplant or not and when. Younger children seem to take organs better; once you have a transplant, you can't be vaccinated. But the diseases themselves would be even more dangerous, too. Being transplanted very young means he'll be back in the game of socialising when he's at the age of socialising. Waiting till he's older means his body is stronger and there might be a greater chance of finding a donor bowel.

And in case you're wondering what kind of bowel we need? We need the same blood group and a baby of the same age to pass away. Another opportunity to make oneself feel bad is lurking… are we waiting for a baby to die for our son to live?

I'm not taking that line of thinking and sinking. Here is how we see it: there is a baby who would have gone regardless of Tuffel's condition. The parents have the opportunity to prevent someone else going through pain by generously releasing the organ. We are not waiting for a death; we are waiting for the generosity of the people who can change Tuffel's – and our – life.

In the meantime, we proceed taking it one day at a time. Which has already led to much deeper presence and enjoyment than I ever thought possible from a situation that can be safely described as challenging.

Here is what my life looks like at the moment: most mornings I get up at 7am, make a spirulina shake (I believe it's good to get the superfood into my system and into the breast milk) that will end up as a green moustache on my face. For some reason Thomas doesn't seem to be attracted to green moustaches. He will let me know most days. I express my milk and have breakfast, then shower. Put clothes and make-up on to cover the moustache. I make a sarnie for lunch, put away all used dishes, devote myself to the endless task of packing the bag with whatever clothes Tuff may need, nappies, wet wipes, whatever else might be on the cards. Then I get out the door and possibly return once for a forgotten item such as a batch of frozen milk for the milk bank or supplies for my next arts and crafts project such as decorating the cot or making a plaster cast of his foot for Grandma that will take me two months to complete.

If it's Wednesday or Friday I go for a quick swim first. Thirty laps in the 25m pool. So picture me rocking up at the pool with five little bottles (around 600ml) of breast milk in tow. " Hi! Good morning, I need your help. Can you store my breast milk in your staff fridge?" The first time I did that I should have taken a picture of the receptionist's face, it was priceless! I explained: "I'd like to go for a swim. I have a baby in hospital and I need a little exercise. However I need to feed that baby and other babies too with my breast milk that I'm bringing in. It needs to be cooled. Would you mind storing it for me please? They are sterile bottles sealed and wrapped nicely in a plastic bag." By now, I have my accomplices and things happen with a "Can you take this for me please?" and a wink and smile. Team Tuffy has expanded all the way to the Clapham Leisure centre.

Today I'm not going to swim as it's raining, and I'm too tired and I'm human, but generally I'm pretty good at taking that little bit of time to myself. Off to hospital between 9am and 10:30. I head home at 7:30pm. I arrive between 7:45 and 8:30pm, cook the lactose and gluten-free dinner we eat at 9pm, clean up and express milk at 22:00 for 30 minutes. In between I try to make a phone call, write or chat with Thomas. Thomas will have worked hard on his new business, an academic tutoring company that uses positive psychology tools practised in America. His business partners are in the States and he's on Skype a lot, researching on the web and concentrating on complicated Excel spreadsheets. Thomas is an entrepreneur throwing himself into the deep end, learning by doing and by reading heaps of books that are piling up on his desk. A real self-starter. Starting a business is risky but, for some people it's the best way forward in life. Thomas would tell you himself that he's pretty unemployable.

However he's struggling with his own bowel issues (which are completely unrelated to Tuffel's). It always makes for interesting conversations. "How are you feeling? How is your stool? How many times? Do you really think it's Crohn's disease? Did you call the doctor? Surely they haven't lost your results again?" Bedtime! Happy days. I get up in the night at 3am to express whilst watching *Horrible Histories* and go back to bed at 4am. Educated, entertained and ever so fatigued. It's a busy day and night, but then again would having a baby at home be so much different? My hat goes off once again to all the mothers of this world for whom endlessly being on call is just what they do…

I'll tell you what really makes me emotional: when a new woman is wheeled into the ward in one of those useless NHS wheelchairs that can only be pulled, not pushed. When I see a woman wheeled in, I get tears in my eyes. Yes, that's how bad that chair is! Nobody wants to be wheeled into the Neonatal Unit. To see a newcomer triggers the pain of the first week. It seems so far away now, so unreal almost. How they told us he wouldn't make it, how Thomas and my mum broke into tears and I just sat there not wanting to buy into it, feeling oddly disconnected. The Westenholzes flying in the next day, my 93-year old great aunt making her way into the hospital and being so deeply affected by seeing him, she wasn't sure it was the right choice. Thomas' dad shaking, having to lean against the wall. When your parents or parents-in-law cry and hold you tight, you know something is really up. How I cried at night in Thomas' arms.

Everyone who is wheeled into the Unit has their own story. And I know it's not the happiest one yet. I just know there is hope in this miracle ward.

I also meet the newbies in the milk expressing room. The mums, obviously – the babies are busy surviving in their incubators. And I'm glad when I meet new mums because I can inject them with a dose of positive mental energy. Lactating is a mental art and hospital is mental; the stress of this setting can make it impossible to lactate, unless you know how to change perspective. And this is where I come in. I have also started making tea for my breastfeeding lady friends to get the milk flowing.

I feel so rich these days. I have everything I need. I have milk galore, I have toys for my boy and I have my wellbeing. Most importantly, I have him and he's thriving. I have a loving relationship and an amazing family and support from my friends. I feel so beautifully held. Is it really a coincidence that Tuffel is doing better than the medics expect? Let's smile together, knowingly (or unknowingly) and keep trusting, praying, loving and hoping for life to unfold its beauty with us.

CHAPTER 7

Are you ready for another miracle?

(4 MONTHS)

I had pointed God to the Neonatal Unit. Seems like someone was listening… Tuffel keeps doing very well. It's been confirmed he's suitable for transplant. But the last couple of weeks were teary. I'd personally like to blame this never-ending grey sky for our low moods, even though I have been perfectly happy in atrocious weather conditions before.

If I were to say that our situation gets to me, most people would respond with an understanding nod. But it's not really the whole truth. It's not the situation that gets to me. The situation is just what it is. Though it's hard, what really gets to me is how I am thinking about it. And how seriously I've been taking this thinking.

I will tell you what triggered my tears of late. We had new neighbours in HDU. A really nice couple with a newborn. I met them coming in from our daily walk. "Oh, that's lucky you can go out," the new dad said. "We haven't had a chance to take her out in a pram yet," he said sadly. "How old is she?" I asked, bewildered. "Three days." Three days? I breathed deeply. Pah! Try 16 weeks and we'll talk. I didn't say that, of course. I asked why they were here. "Well, she had an obstruction in her bowel, we were rushed in and they broke through the obstruction surgically." I could see he was convinced he had a tough story.

If there were a dial indicating the severity of one's bowel issue, they'd sit at the opposite end from us. We would have loved for Tuffel to only have a bowel obstruction! I shouldn't say that. I am far too spiritually evolved to compare my situation with others…

When he heard that the worst-case scenario of what they were enduring was occupying the space right next to them, you could feel his inside slump. I'm competitive. So I slumped even lower. How unfair is life? Why didn't Tuffel just have that? Instead we have the odd one out, never-seen-anything-like-it saga. I know I am reacting to my thoughts and thoughts aren't real unless you buy into them. I certainly spent my mental cash on a variety of dark thoughts. I spent almost as much mental cash as the Greeks spent Euros. Well, not quite, but at least it sounds like I still follow the news.

On a lighter note, Thomas finally had an MRI scan to investigate his own bowel issues (he had waited for two months), the contrasting drugs leaving him feeling horrid. Or maybe he felt horrid because we realised that he really has kept on losing weight. He's faded to 60kg. That's 9.4 stone for those of you who prefer to get stoned, weight wise. I love that weight still gets measured in 'stone'. How heavy is a stone? Two rocks, of course. If we measure weight in stone, we should refer to length in 'strings'. How long is the cupboard? Three pieces of string long and two strings wide. Now that's what I call a good-sized cupboard.

But I ask you: how long is a piece of string?

So yes, nine stones and four pebbles is Thomas' current weight – that's not much above me. He stands at six smelly feet tall. Thomas needs help, fast.

No amount of food seems to be helping. The doctors suspect Crohn's disease. Crohn's is a chronic inflammation of the small intestine. Sixty per cent of sufferers will lose part of that bowel due to the disease. I spoke to one sufferer living on TPN (that's the same artificial nutrition that Tuffel gets) only a few months ago. Do we really need another incurable bowel disease in this family? Seriously. What is this shit with my men and their bowels?

So that's the situation at present. I'm not finding it easy. If we measured ease in pieces of cake (Poc) I'd say we are definitely in the negative. This doesn't feel like a very cakey situation. Minus 10 Poc. No cream.

So are you ready for a miracle? Because we are. We so are. It's been brewing for a while and it's becoming more real now… we are planning on taking Tuffel home.

Yes, you read that correctly: We are taking him **HOME!**

Pre-transplant, with all his machines.

Yes, yes, yes, there are many hurdles. He needs to be off his TPN for 10 hours a day. I remember being able to take him out for one hour, then two. Now we are at five! During that time, he has to balance his own blood sugar levels. He will need one or two operations to change his plumbing. We'll need training and a qualification to handle TPN so we know what to do when the various pumps alarm. There won't be a nurse to sort it out. Whatever. I'm going to get my son! Oh, and another minor detail. We need a home. Our flat is too small for his machinery and supplies, they say.

Our flat is already too full. "Is that where you got his name from?" asked my hospital mummy friend Sarah. Too-full-Tuffel.

So we are buying a house. We are looking for three to four bedrooms in a nice area, with a garden, close to a park and transport. To stay in our area, we need almost £1 million. We wouldn't get a mortgage for half of that – so I've been arranging viewings in the less glamorous parts of South London. It's amazing what the introduction "I have a boy in hospital whom I can take out when I've got a house with enough space for his medical supplies. What can you show me?" does to estate agents. Some of them even call back! If you happened to see a big umbrella with two people under it bickering that "this isn't like Clapham", it was probably Thomas and me house hunting.

Finding a house is somewhere between one and -100 Poc. It started at an enthusiastic 4 Poc and three parts cream and went down to -11 in about three weeks.

However, from the perspective of my breast pump, this has been an interesting journey to say the least. It has seen many more places now. I could do a YouTube clip tracking the whereabouts of my little breast pump. Pumping in Sydenham. What an inspiring title for a movie. Except I can't be bothered. It's no wonder I've been tired. My days are long and the nights are short and in between there is kind of a lot going on. In addition, a silent dread about life after hospital has crept into my mind. They do give us a lot of support... what will I do on my own?

So I joined the grey clouds above and cried. And then I prayed – please help me. I cannot do this anymore! It's all too much. Show me the way out. A prayer isn't limited to a religious ritual. A prayer is a wish expressed to the greater intelligence behind life.

The next morning Thomas and I both went to hospital to see our beautiful baby boy. The best thing one can do when weighed down by the inner darkness is to face reality. We have had dark thoughts about our grim and isolated future, worried about all the things we were told it could bring. We've been told: "People have suicidal thoughts," or, "It's hard looking after a baby like this," or, "Forget about working; this is literally full-time." With this in my mind, I get stressed, distressed and tired. But luckily these thoughts all dissolve in the presence of love.

There he was, the Tuffmeister, in his little beige bouncing chair with the dangling plush toys merrily moving above his cute little head. And he looked at us and smiled. For the first time. Mouth open and eyes shining. Tuffel's smile. The world stopped and became a happy place again. A happy place I'd like to call home. With a solid score of 50Poc and five cream puffs. Tuffel is taking us home.

And that is another miracle.

CHAPTER 8

Amazing Grace

(4 MONTHS)

Amazing Grace
how sweet thy sound
that saved a wretch like me
I once was lost but now am found
was blind, but now I see

When I sang this to our little group in the morgue, my voice broke. I was off pitch but I didn't want to stop. I prayed for spirit to lift me through this. After all, I was singing for Grace. I started again and relaxed as I felt my voice carrying the sound, resonating with the love and soul I had intended to share in that moment. Singing was the best way for me to communicate. This was important to me. I didn't have words or defined feelings; I needed the sound of my voice to express. I could see in her parents' eyes that it meant more to them than any of us could ever understand.

Grace joined our ward having been born prematurely at 30 weeks and 5 days weighing only 1.23kg with a heart condition and something was up with her bowel too- she had an atresia in the Duodenum which was fixed (though surgery) after she was born. She was very sweet and looked so cosy tucked up in her mum Sarah's bosom, or under her dad Steve's shirt. Kangaroo care means the little one gets as much body contact as possible, which helps them develop outside the womb. Mum's heartbeat is something familiar and soothing. I'm such a fan of kangaroo care I suppose I just took it to the next level with my legendary topless sessions. Kangaroo care is the British version of skin-to-skin care. I could never be that discreet.

Little Grace was always dressed in the most adorable pink outfits, and I could see Tuffy eyeing up her lovingly decorated cot with its plethora of soft toys and one of those mobiles that is pleasant rather than offensive to our senses. Grace had very loving parents. I enjoyed our chats over cuddles with our little ones. Other mums meet for coffee; here in the Neonatal Ward we do simultaneous cuddle sessions if we're lucky. Not all children are that much loved and wanted.

Needless to say, Grace did very well and grew stronger. Sarah was unable to breast feed Grace as it was important that all her feeds were accurately measured based on her weight. I was always informed with the latest news as we had become a lovely little group: Claire, Elaine, Sarah and me. Sharing chats, cups of tea and the ups and downs of our kids. Even though we all have friends, nobody will ever understand the hospital situation as much as someone who is in it themselves.

Grace had her first heart operation and recovered well. After only three months it was decided she could go home. How we envied them and at the same time were thrilled, of course. The rest of us didn't know how long we'd have to stay. Nobody can tell with our babies. Sarah and Steve went nursery shopping and got a pram, changing mat, nappy bin and all the nursery furniture in preparation of Grace's homecoming to Haywards Heath. Knowing them, they didn't save on it – they wanted the best for their little long-awaited princess. We were all sharing in their excitement.

But the next day, little Grace took a sudden turn for the worse and had to undergo a second heart operation. She recovered well and all was set for her to go home.

And when I came into the hospital on Monday morning, Claire was there, in tears. Elaine was crying, too. What the heck had happened? Grace had died. I remember the shock. I had witnessed a few deaths by this time, but this was different again. Grace was fine and she was meant to go home that week! How cruel does life get? Sarah and Steve were devastated; we didn't know what to say but we didn't have to say anything. We just cried together.

They invited us to see her in the morgue. As uncomfortable as that invitation could be, it was certainly not one we would decline. Thomas came too. They keep the bodies refrigerated and when you have your time, they very carefully arrange the room adequately. When we came in, we saw Grace in a cot with her cuddly toys around her. She looked rosy and beautiful. No more cables, no more lines, no annoyances.

Sarah picked the stiff cold corpse out of the cot and held her in her arms. That's when I sang. It felt right, but boy that was hard. I mustn't let my mind run into the tears. Easier said than done.

Sarah offered her to us to hold, too. Which was a hugely trusting and generous gesture. But I couldn't. That was simply too much for me. I politely declined, feeling dreadful. The last thing I wanted was to cause an awkward situation. But we all gave her a kiss. And that to me was very uncomfortable too. Kissing a corpse is so far out my comfort zone. I didn't want to be disrespectful. Death is so strange and mysterious and a dead body is such an unfamiliar experience to me. I felt so exposed to my discomfort in all this. But I couldn't be bothered to go into my personal feelings. This was way bigger. I kissed the cold cheek of baby Grace. Rest in peace little angel.

The funeral was arranged a few weeks later and was such a sad, beautiful, respectful ceremony. Nurses, doctors, friends and family formed a 100-strong congregation.

Steve and Sarah raised money for the ward in Grace's honour, to be used for a new incubator with a plaque in honour of little Grace and her friends. I was stunned by their resilience and generosity. Having just lost their daughter, they had every right to run from the hospital never to come back. To be angry at the world and its unfairness. Instead, they gave thanks. Thanks for all the help they had received. I have so much respect for them. Sarah came back to the ward to be with us; it must have felt so empty to sit in the hallway alone. You're only allowed into the rooms to see your child. No cross-visiting is allowed, due to infection risk. We knew each other's kids via photos (unless we were allocated to the same room).

The day of the funeral had been grey and rainy. The pink balloons with messages of love for Grace couldn't really take off – the wind and rain brought them right down, reminding us of the fact that rituals and ceremonies are a lovely idea but they are not what define our love. Grace had brought a lot of sweetness – and grace to our lives. We are saddened that her own life was so short. But we all agreed with Sarah that – it was better than suffering, and "enough is enough". When they had tried to resuscitate her, running out of access points, the doctors were drilling holes into her shin bone. It must have been a terrible ordeal, but their job is to do everything possible. Sarah said: "Look, if we are going to lose her, can we leave this and can I just cuddle her?" She cut the suffering short – the strongest and most courageous thing a mother could do.

Amazing Sarah, showing us amazing Grace.

Life is not fair. Envy has no place. May the Grace we were blessed to experience lead us to a gentler and more gracious way of being in the world.

CHAPTER 9

We could all use a lesson in self-soothing

(4 MONTHS)

Prince Tuffel the Great has mastered the art of self-soothing, a skill invaluable for life. I can recommend self-soothing to anyone – thumb sucking optional. I've recently had the opportunity to learn a lot from Tuffel's ability to calm himself. Lately, I've felt stretched beyond my limit. Off my Poc Richter scale.

The tension between Thomas and me has been increasing dramatically. Arguments erupting on a daily basis, tears flowing and frustration driving us to the edge. We make mountains out of molehills. But having said that, I've come to the conclusion that it's just an attempt to make things bigger and better. After all, nobody travels to climb a molehill. Mountains are awe-inspiring. They are worthy of attention. So we blow up our issues to finally get the attention we crave. Or maybe it's just me?

Except the mountains of our perceived problems aren't that pretty. They are just petty.

"I hate that you don't clean your dishes." (me)

"I do clean them."

"But not when we agree you'll do them. So if you leave things out, by the time you do intend to clear them I will have used the kitchen twice. I need it clean and hygienic now."

"There are lots of things you don't do. You're totally messy."

"I think you are messy. Look at all your stuff that's been lying around for months."

"Oh yeah? Your stuff has been here for years and I'm sick of it."

"You have football goals in their original packaging you've never used and will never use in the middle of the hallway. I hate that you expect me to clean and cook and shop. That's not what I signed up for. Why should I do all of it?"

"I work non-stop without breaks from morning to night, I don't even get dressed sometimes. No, after 10-12 hours I am not up for more chores. I have headaches and stomach aches most days. But I don't moan about it. You are so spoilt. We can swap any day. You make the money for the family and I learn to take care of Tuff and cook. Fine with me. At least you do what you love every day. I need some time to live my own life."

"I want you to do what you love and make the money with that."

"Me too, but it's not realistic right now."

"But you play football, and PlayStation, meet friends and let me do all the work at home. I am in hospital all day. Then I work, and I express milk, which takes an hour each time. I don't have any time to myself. I also arrange the house viewings. What else?"

"You chose to be a mum."

Ugly visions of lonely futures play out and my fears of separation, rooted in childhood, aim straight at my weak spots, sinking their claws into the flesh of my nerves. When tied up in these emotions, I lose sight of reality. I lose sight of wisdom. Wisdom that would tell me that we're okay, just tired. That Thomas loves me and that I love him and the rest is pretty secondary. I'm not hearing this wisdom. The nasty feelings feel real, and the thoughts around it feel real. I forget they are just thoughts. Because, can't you see, I am having a real problem.

I've asked the girls. Seems like many young families find themselves arguing more after a baby comes along. When we ask why some houses are up for sale we hear that the couple has split up. After baby. The house half done up. Gulp.

What on earth does having a lovely new addition in life do to make you argue? We should be happy! Especially us. We know how precious life is. What is this about destroying the good times like this? Stupid! Stupid. Let's not do it anymore. Enough of this silliness. The number of times we've said that…To be fair we have also stopped it numerous times. But like a fire partially smothered, it just flares up again. I could feel that the underlying issue was not resolved. But I couldn't figure out what it was.

House hunting must be taking its toll on us. I don't get it. I love looking at houses! So it's obvious, it's HIM! Why does he have to make it a miserable experience? I put so much effort into it and he brings his foul mood. I'm not a victim at all… only 100 per cent.

We have such original topics to argue about. Here is the short version – I bet you've never heard arguments along these lines:

"Can you clear the table from your papers please, as you promised?"

"I never promised."

"Yes, you did."

"Stop bullying me; you are so annoying."

"Oh shut up and do what you said you would. I'm tired of your excuses!"

"Leave me alone – you're too much to be around!"

Which eventually boils over to this more explosive version – I have added subtitles:

"You said you'd do the washing today." (Subtext: Why do I even have to mention that?)

"I've really had enough of your criticising." (Subtext: f*** off)

"I'm not criticising you." (I'm just telling you what to do because you don't seem to be able to do that yourself, you moron)

"Just leave me alone!" (I will not talk about it nor will I do whatever I may have said I would, which I never cared about in the first place and even less so, now that you reminded me of it!)

But when push comes to shove, we do stick together. We go through thick and thin. It just seems we're a bit thick about it sometimes. Meanwhile, I mentioned Thomas was getting rather thin, right?

On Thursday the 17th of May Thomas dragged himself home from football feeling worse than ever, his friend Sebastian at his side. "Call an ambulance – I need to go to hospital," he said. He'd had a particularly shitty day. After eight visits to the loo, dehydration and stomach cramps had left him in agony. I suggested calling a cab. Ten minutes later he didn't want to go to hospital anymore. "What are they going to do for me? They never help me when I try to get treatment." Then, as he bent forward again, I could see he was really struggling. "Let's go to hospital if you feel that bad," I offered. He agreed.

Two minutes later he started arguing about it again. "I don't know where my things are, I don't want to go." I packed a bag, called the cab and took him to A&E. Confusion is a symptom of severe dehydration and it's certainly not Thomas' usual behaviour. "Why are we going? It makes no sense," he argued back and forth for the duration of the ride. I couldn't wait to get him seen. When it was our turn, they agreed he needed fluids and by 1:30am he was admitted to a ward. I had spent all day and then all evening in hospital. I was at the end of my tether. Two men in hospital. And if that was not enough, Tuffy was going to have an operation the next morning. To put it in Tuffel's words: Whaaaaaeeea!!!

2am: I went back to the Neonatal Unit, where I can always find company and compassion, and dissolved into tears.

The wonderful sister in charge offered me a room for the night (with a view of Big Ben) and I settled for three hours of sleep before I received a wake-up text: "They are not giving me fluids. Please come ASAP." It was the classic NHS hospital nightmare. The fluids had been prescribed in A&E, he had been advised not to eat and drink. Up in the ward, some doctor put Thomas "on hold" without communicating why. The nurses were not allowed to act; the ward round was scheduled between 8am and 9am. I pushed several times to get someone in. Admitted for dehydration, they had left him to dry out all night. Thomas had rung the bell only for someone to come and turn it off without even speaking to him. As Tuffel would say: Waaaaaaheeha haaaeee!!!*&@!

What a different world from our fabulous Neonatal Unit. Our nurses and doctors actually care. They listen. They believe in better. They keep training; they communicate and allow us to be part of discussions. They disclose and explain. Over in the adult ward, it's a different ball game. No one seems to want to discuss; they speak over your head when they speak at all; meals are skipped and understaffing is prominent. To the extent that they sent him home four days later because no one could see him anyway, so he'd be better off going home and waiting for his outpatient appointment. There was only one gastroenterologist working for two hospitals and he was overwhelmed.

But before that, I found myself running between wards. We needed to get Tuffel ready for his operation: his nutrition would no longer be pumped through a tiny line in his arm, but though a bigger line funnelled under his skin entering the blood stream at neck level called a Broviac, Hickman or simply central line. I love the term 'central line'. I will never look at the London Underground system in the same way.

Why are they doing this? Because it's a more durable line. But medical resoning aside, he will be able to wear clothes without leaving one arm undressed. And I like the idea of using both sleeves in a garment. What a novelty. And now for the extra bonus: with this new line, during his hours off he will be wireless. Wireless!

From a fashion perspective, the day of the operation was a real gem. My two men were sporting the same outfits in very different sizes. It was my Monsoon dream (mummy and daughter in the same glittery princess-style garments) gone ape shape. But still, Gok Wan eat your heart out. You couldn't get this gear on the high street if you tried.

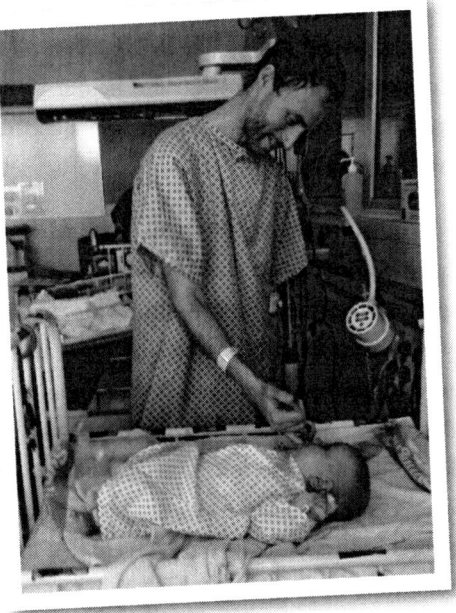

As is typical, the operation got delayed. Tuffy had been nil by mouth since early morning. But only I got nervous about it. This clever little boy just sucked his thumb and slept. He did not complain. He seems to do important things so beautifully. At the last assessment at King's Hospital they told me it would be good if he could sleep through his cat scan at 11:35. As if you can make a baby sleep on command. But he mustn't move for the camera. Sure, not to worry, I'll just tell my baby that. What are these people thinking?

I whispered to him that it would be good if he could please sleep for the scan. Might as well try. But he was wide awake when I pushed him in the pram and had him on the breast. When they called me in they asked me to take him off the boob and place him on the scanning plate. I expected protest – babies tend not to like being taken off the boob. Well, who does, really? But what did he do? Came off and just slipped into a snooze. And woke up when the scan was done, five minutes later!

I took him down to theatre at 4pm. That's when reality hit. He was going under general anaesthetics. The implications were explained; I signed the consent form. You know when they say 'sign your life away'? Well, that's basically what we do when we sign the form. Tears welling up. Yes, I'm okay. No, I don't have any questions. Let's just do this. I gave him a kiss, they gave the injection and ushered me out of the room. "Okay mummy he's sleeping; you can go now." His eyes had been rolling upwards, were still open – I had to trust it would be fine.

One and a half hours later I got the call that he was awake and everything had gone smoothly. We took him upstairs, and the little star launched straight into a breastfeed. He was sucking away as if the operation had never happened.

Meanwhile, Thomas was getting more and more upset about the lack of treatment, the world in general and his whole situation. I didn't want to argue with that, but it was incredibly hard to bear. I'm also not sure how that would help anyone's tummy trouble, but I could feel it was the wrong time to mention that part. My friend, Sarah-Louise, came – what great timing – and brought him food. Ironically, hospitals don't cater for lactose intolerance, not even for gastroenterological patients. So they'd rather have them get really ill while they're in the hospital's care? I could see that logic in a privatised environment – what a great money-spinner. But for the NHS? Completely counterproductive.

The next day I went to a house viewing – call me mad, but this place looked too good to be missed – picked a few bits up for Thomas' birthday, cooked two meals that wouldn't waste away in a hospital room without a fridge whilst expressing breast milk, then hurried to St Thomas'. I was so proud of how I had multitasked. And glad my blood pressure wasn't measured that day. But instead of being showered with admiration, I got a right dressing down. Thomas had been hungrily pacing the room for hours and didn't quite appreciate the home-cooked food. He would have preferred things more quickly. I suppose a lot of things came together for him to get so angry. Possibly being put into isolation and told he couldn't see his son tipped him over the edge. To cut an ugly conversation short, I left the room and was told not to come back for the next few days. I knew he wouldn't mean it for long. But I had no more resources left to let it bounce off me. I was done.

Tears flooding, I curled up in the corner next to Tuffy's cot. I don't deserve this! I felt like a beaten wife stuck between hell and a bad place. I was too tired to think any sense and just felt awful. My nurses lent me their ears, hearts and support. I have friends in the Unit and two cups of tea and five colourful Jubilee macaroons later, the world looked a little brighter again. You can't really stay miserable with theatrically coloured cakes. Gold, silver and copper! Plus, I have the most wonderful little boy looking at me.

Thomas would come round again. Ideally, before his birthday. Which was the next day. I had planned a surprise for him: having involved the nurses in charge, I had been granted special permission to take Tuffy to the park with the whole family. I'd had first-aid training (in secret) and was so excited. Now with Thomas in hospital, those plans had been thwarted. Well, my Tomtom didn't even want to see me. I did a lot of breathing, crying and feeling exceptionally tired and drained that day.

I don't give up when it comes to making life special. So… I bought party decorations. Luckily, by that evening Thomas and I had a heart-to-heart. He does always come round; I wish I could remember that when it's all kicking off. The next morning I turned his ugly side room without a view into London's premier party location.

With a big Happy Birthday banner and stars dangling, the whole family ended up celebrating, with lactose and gluten-free cake made by Thomas' Aunty Inge. Thomas was wearing his sexy hospital robe in faded orange. Irresistible.

If we were cowboys, we'd now be riding off into the sunset. No sunset on the horizon for now – we'll stay put on a hospital bed at St. Thomas' Hospital, gazing into each other's eyes.

CHAPTER 10

Oh, such a perfect day

(5 MONTHS)

Another weekend in the Neonatal Unit approached. Tuffy, the big fish in his pond of newborn tadpoles, was looking up at our consultant, Alan. I've enjoyed many forward-thinking conversations with this bright-eyed Irish medic. "Have you been out much?" he wants to know. "No, we are still restricted to hospital grounds, but we'd love to change that."

"Where would you want to go?" enquired Alan in his gorgeous Irish accent.

"Home."

"Home?"

"Home."

"But what if you need care?"

"We live 10 minutes away by car. We could get back in a flash."

"Do you have a car?"

"No. But we can rent one."

"What about a car seat?" I love how he cares about the details.

Oh, we have a car seat. Black and turquoise. The car seat is what you bring to hospital to take your baby home in. We've had it for ages. When I'm having a 'down day', I start to drown in jealousy when I see men carrying them into hospital, looking sheepish in the lift. The Postnatal Ward is located opposite the Neonatal Unit. Go on then, rub it in. The members of the Neonatal Club all share this little nagging sense of envy.

The car seat: our symbol of hope. I refused to get rid of ours.

It had been sitting in our flat, now a dumping ground for coats, for the last five months. That was the best thing to do with it. Especially as we don't have a coat rack in our flat – it's not that I wouldn't want one, but living in a rented flat in England means you can't just put things up. You can't hammer a nail into the wall. When we buy a place, I will put nails and coat racks on every wall that hasn't asked for one. I will make wall-art out of nails. I will have to buy coats for all the new racks. I will hang my car seat up on a coat rack just to prove the point.

"Tuffel doesn't really have any urgent medical needs; let me see what I can do," said Alan. "He just looks *bralliant – ameezin*," he concluded, before continuing his ward round, a twinkle in his eye. On Friday afternoon Alan resurfaced. "Right, I've got it all cleared. This has never happened in the history of the Neonatal Unit. You can go home. Please come back an hour before his TPN goes up."

I gasped for air in excitement: the coat seat will become a car seat! My coats will have to lie on the floor for the day. Thank you, Alan.

With my 'outlaws' over (they would be my in-laws if Thomas got his act together and a very nice ringaling), we'd have a real family weekend. None of this two-people-at-the-cot-at-once malarkey (Neonatal Unit rules), while two of us sit in reception, drowning our sorrows with tea served in environmentally controversial polystyrene cups as we wait our turn. We could have proper cups of course. I actually bought two sets of cutlery for the parents' room in the Unit. They disappeared within 10 days. Though environmentally friendlier, I don't want to lose my temper over missing crockery. That's not good for the immediate environment, either.

Cups and cutlery aside: this is the day we go to our home! We'll all be together. How cosy to sit on the couch. It's interesting how a crammed London one-bedroom flat can suddenly become a family idyll.

How good can life get?

Even the gloomy weather made an exception to celebrate the occasion. How wonderful to fit the car seat adapters to the buggy, the car seat slotting in perfectly. Tuffel looked great in it. *Ameezin*. Just *bralliant*.

Everyone got excited for us and waved us good-bye. Imogen, one of my favourite nurses, turned away quickly as she got tears in her eyes. "Have a great day!" Thank you, we will.

Sitting on the sofa instead of an NHS chair does make a difference. Being served olive bread with hummus and prosciutto while breastfeeding, now *that* is what I call the good life. And then my personal highlight – cuddling up in bed. Thomas, Tuffel and I. The family moment. After five long months. So worth it. Then, we went for a walk on Clapham Common. Grandma, Grandpa, Daddy, Mummy and baby Tuffel. Just another happy family on a Saturday afternoon. Music was playing at the bandstand and we enjoyed a cappuccino at the park café, surrounded by scooters and buggies. You'd see us, just like any other family and you'd never know how super special this was. I wonder what people did think, seeing us sitting there with tears our eyes.

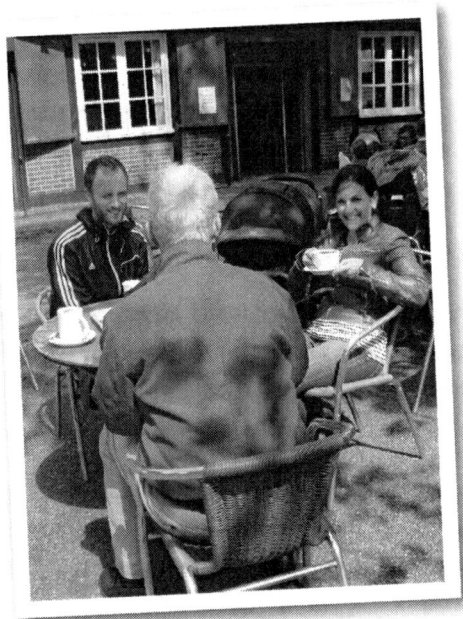

Oh, such a perfect day

As much as I had been getting excited at the prospect of taking Tuff home, I had been secretly dreading it, too. Without the safety of the hospital, how would I get on? Without the help of the many staff, would I cope?

So that afternoon I just got on with life and did Tuffy's afternoon cares in the comfort of my own home. I had brought the equipment and to make a short story even shorter, it was so easy! He was so relaxed and seemed to just be happy where he was. My worries dissolved into thin air. Maybe a little fart. I did smell something. Might have been the stoma bag. Who cares?

When we returned to the Unit, we were greeted like long-lost friends. To be so welcomed is just wonderful. Our first flight from the nest was a complete success. Soon we'd take off for good...

To make good things better, Thomas and I decided to tackle our relationship issues in the most efficient way: counselling. But no, that didn't work out. The counsellor arrived 35 minutes late without apology and didn't even seem to feel the tension in the room. Thomas had taken the afternoon off work to do this session and some Tuffel-care training and none of it was happening. He wasn't impressed with that. So she stated he must be very stressed and overwhelmed about time. "How does that feel?" she probed, and strangely enough, Thomas doesn't like being labelled with a problem he doesn't have. Clearly, she had the time problem, not him!

So, instead of the 'psycho babble', I got a cleaner and that seemed to kill two birds with one stone: (A) It put a stop to our ongoing arguments and (B) we have a clean flat! And that's what we call value for money.

It's important to invest in one's relationship. Thomas recognised that in just the right way and to acknowledge my contribution to the family and give me a lovely surprise, he booked me a day at the spa. Claire (my new friend from the Unit) and I took a whole day off from being hospital mummies and enjoyed ourselves thoroughly. We had a massage, used the steam room, relaxed to meditation tapes in a dark and comfortable room, ate beautiful food we didn't have to stand in a queue to purchase or have to warm in a microwave. Expressing milk has never been so glamorous as sitting in a spa lounge with a fine cup of tea. This little breast pump of mine does get around.

What I am learning is that it's not all about how life is treating you, but how we treat life – and which spa treatments to have in life. Full-body massage, anyone?

CHAPTER 11

All change! Wards, tubes and moods

(6 MONTHS)

My American sister, Rhonda, (I spent seven months in the States with a host family when I was 16) has the cutest little boy, Jacob, who has a male doll.

Yes, there are male dolls. Not many apart from Ken – and he is only kind of male. Barbie and Ken got divorced in 2004. It was announced by their spokesperson. Some say it was a publicity stunt, but according to Mattel, the spark had gone. Divorced Barbie now comes with Ken's house, Ken's car… bad joke – got it from the internet.

Anyway, cute little Jacob named his doll Tuffel, and he makes him play football. Now that is cool.

I am touched by the way that people who know us now care and share…

Rich Litvin (one of my favourite coaches) and his wife Monique DeBose have Kaleo, who is 4 months older than Tuffel, and they recently took part in a walk for sick children in LA. They walked for Baby Tuffel.

And the multitalented Sonja Morgenstern sent me this cartoon titled Tuffel's first date:

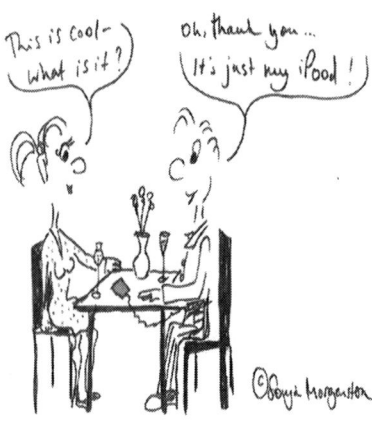

I'm thrilled with the impact Tuffel is making on people's lives, and that he's touched so many people around the world.

Meanwhile, back at the ranch, it seems Tuffel has outstayed his welcome in the Neonatal Unit. After five months, a place has become available at the nearby Evelina Children's Hospital. To make this incredible story even more incredible, our names, Thomas and Evelyne, are matched with the hospitals our son will have called home: St. Thomas' and Evelina.

We have been desperate for more space. The High Dependency Unit is crammed. But it has become home.

Since our successful first day trip, we've been allowed out on a regular basis. Tuffy is by now given eight hours of wireless freedom a day, which means that he can keep his blood sugar levels stable for eight hours – I don't know if I can do that! And because he is able to do that, most of his time is spent outside of the ward anyway.

We were prepared for him to wait for a few years for this, but admittedly we've gotten used to this very quickly in the best possible way: we spend a lot of time out pretending to be normal. I can't go to baby groups due to infection risks – I cannot afford to bring a virus into the environment of highly vulnerable preterm babies – but I can be in the park or at home, or see a friend. I mustn't be in crowded places or with anyone who isn't feeling well.

And the time has come: we were told to transfer to the children's hospital. We didn't want to go. We love the nurses and the doctors. Yvonne, the surgical nurse we're so fond of, has started teaching us about TPN (Tuffel's 'space food' and how to administer it). I may not need to cook for my son, but his meals are high maintenance to say the least. Sir prefers it sterile. I feel like hugging Yvonne every time I see her. She was also our first contact when we got the news that we'd have to spend some time at the hospital after birth. She explained what that meant and took Thomas to see the Unit. I couldn't take it back then. The idea of seeing babies in incubators with tubes and wires was too much to handle for my pregnant self. I remember drinking a cup of very sweet tea while waiting for Thomas to return from his mission. I was so surprised when he said, "Babe, it's actually quite nice there. The nurses are really friendly and they have time for you; they smile and they are laughing. You wouldn't believe it, but it's a good atmosphere. Our baby will be in good hands."

He was right.

I feel like reminiscing now that this hard but special time is coming to an end: Fabiana is one of our favourite nurses here. She calls Tuffel her boyfriend. So does Jade. Jade is Caribbean with a huge smile and a massive heart. She gave him a hand knitted yellow and green Teddy and signed it "From Jade, your first love". Fabiana is from Brazil. She claims that, as she is younger, surely Tuffel would want to be with her. She's been with us on a day trip to King's and called it her date. Tuffel is taking her out.

Ruwenna and Zeni are two more of my top stars. They are from the Philippines. I love how neat they are. I can tell when they've been on shift because the sheets are straight and the cot is organised, and possibly the cupboard too. Ruwenna has been known to say, "You are so cute, I will put you in my rucksack and take you hooome." I'd like to put her into my rucksack and let her loose on my flat! Zeni will always be remembered for her interrogating: "Tuffeeeel my freeend, why you so tired, eeh? What you dooo last night? You serenade somebahdy? Eh, Tuffeeel? I'm jokiiiin!"

Then there's Heather, who always comes up with a new way of hanging toys in places Tuffy can see them. She's my arts and crafts nurse. She's always cheerful and so friendly. British, so no fun accent, but she comes up with cool ways of cutting plasters – she always thinks of possible improvements. It is thanks to Heather that they stopped pricking Tuffy's heels twice a day for blood. Blood-sugar testing is a shift routine, but when there is no need, let's change the system! And so she did. She also created the special Tuffel sheet, which unified the way we were measuring his stats. And thanks to her I don't get frontal poos all over me anymore. She introduced stoma bags, which ended a lot of his annoyance at life and keeps me smelling much nicer, too.

His outputs and inputs are confusing – when you see a kid with tubes like Tuffy has, it's usually to get food in. But in his case, it's to get food out. When the continuing care nurse (who will help us by organising a care package from the council, so that we will have nurses to help out at home for some hours) came to assess us, you could see she was mentally trying to picture the anatomy. She asked: "So you put things out of the feeding tube and feed it into the stoma – does he have an exit?" And I said: "Yes. It's called an arsehole." I know it was patronising, but I couldn't resist.

And there's 'Aunty Jenny', who's now a children's rep in Egypt to take a sabbatical from nursing – she was special. When we met her we thought, 'Gee, what a ditzy blonde'. Northern accent, high-pitched voice. The only thing missing was the heels and a sexy nursing gown. Jenny would wear the outfit if given half a chance. Sadly, they have to wear scrubs. Or, if we were to call a spade a spade, purple pyjamas. What we loved was how she chatted away to all the babies as well as being a highly skilled, extremely friendly, superb and wonderful nurse. You should have seen Tuffy's face when she came round. We all miss Jenny at the Unit. Jenny, you are amazing.

Marcia felt like a grandmother to us. She was so gentle with him whilst inserting tubes, and gave me hope of breastfeeding him one day. The warmth and smiles make all the difference in an environment of distress. They are what turns the nightmare into a surprisingly rich experience.

My German nurse, Nicole, went back to Germany. Funnily, she's from a place close to my home. She was efficient, friendly and professional. I didn't want her to leave. She's German in the best possible sense.

And there's Keith, too. Long live the male nurses! Keith, in his spare time, volunteers for St John Ambulance. So if you are at a festival, falling ill, you might meet him one day too. He's a geeky type – he has a pet rabbit. Keith is the guy who will in all innocence proclaim: "I'll be your dirty nurse," and I'd repeat it and then he'd blush. In nursing, the person who isn't sterile is called the 'dirty nurse'. Keith is so innocent I'd have to explain to him what a dirty nurse does in my world. His classic quote was asking Heather whether he could "plunge his syringe into her driver". Call me bad, but I enjoyed making him blush. Again.

I could go on and on. I'm telling you, the people who have cared for Tuffel are incredible.

I feel I've made real friends. I always thought I'd meet the amazing people of this world at the heights of success. You know, famous people – producers, musicians, actors – people with stories and character. But I've met them here in the Neonatal Unit. The nurses are such wonderful human beings.

I'm in awe of the team in Neonatal – and the drive to keep learning and training and helping these little darlings. Most nurses are passionate about their jobs. How else could they work 12 hour shifts, day and night? I love the amount of care and time they have for us. I love that they taught me so much about nursing my son. I couldn't imagine a life without this intensive care family.

From being told that we were going to have to move soon to packing our bags for Evelina, it was just three days. Then we were gone. With a big trolley and two bin bags of breast milk bottles that fell off the trolley halfway. The joy!

Everyone agrees that Evelina Hospital is much better for a child. There is more space, more freedom. There are play specialists (Bekka, in particular, rocks) and other children, and colours and noises. There is even a fold-out mattress I can use to stay overnight. You can chill there with your homies, or Nala the golden retriever – one of the therapy dogs who regularly visits the children in the hospital.

But there are hundreds of new nurses who are busy with patients and unfamiliar with the special case of Mr T which had the consequences of discomfort, X-rays, and denying him food for hours or days on end. It wasn't funny to say the least. The first two weeks are too hard to repeat here. All the tears and desperation until late at night – and I'm not even talking about Tuffel. I was so upset. New doctors, new consultants, new everyone.

How many times I talked them through how to do his cares, how important it is that he receives his TPN on time as blood sugar levels HAVE to be maintained and how many times it got ignored, or lost in translation. I will mention Sheryl here as our angel nurse. She took charge and really got stuck into trying to sort things out for us. Nurses work in shifts, so we had a new one almost every day. Sheryl made notes that too often weren't read and briefed staff about what was important, only for me to come in and find it hadn't been done. I pity the hospital staff (and there would be a few) who have gotten to know a more highly strung version of me. I missed my peaceful, happy self.

It reminded me of the days we spent at King's Hospital for the transplant assessment. Where they didn't have the supplies I needed for his cares. It was such a surprise to me that two hospitals in the same country, the same city, could be so different. This is, in effect, was just another building within the same hospital. They are even using differently shaped milk bottles here. I rest my case.

Days drew out longer and my self-care routine went out the window. I just couldn't trust they'd get it right and I didn't want to get Tuffel into more discomfort than necessary. It's no wonder I got sick. I literally got sick and tired of it.

CHAPTER 12

Coping and hoping

(6 MONTHS)

Once healthy again, we headed back down the long hallways to the parents' room at the Neonatal Unit. My home. It's the strangest thing to come 'home' when you're no longer living there. I missed my friends, the nurses, Claire and Casper. We had spent a long time together and a whole book could easily be written about their intense journey. I wanted to see how he was doing but, as Tuffy was no longer a patient of the ward, they wouldn't let me back inside with Tuffel. I hoped to catch Claire in the parents' room, if my timing coincided with her tea break – this could happen. But she too was juggling milk production, medical care and doctors with being present for her precious boy.

My breast milk for donation was slowly filling up the fridges in our ward at Evelina. Slowly, because too many bottles been wasted by nurses taking it out too early, defrosting too much at once or fridges failing overnight. Sometimes a door was left open and litres of white liquid gold would go to waste.

What was left, I took to the milk bank at the Neonatal Unit. I don't envy the nurse in charge of counting my milk. It's freezing cold and there is lots of it. Breast milk is a precious commodity and when it's not given to a baby on the ward, it is sold to other hospitals for around £100 per litre. But first it runs through a sterilising process, so every bottle has to be marked with name of donor and date of production. Even frozen, it only has a shelf life of six months.

I had been quite ambitious trying to break the record for most milk donated. When I say ambitious, I mean slightly obsessed and then frustrated. My lovely 36B bouncing Buddhas were doing their best, but I felt quite defeated at 40 litres. I know that's a lot, but losing milk to sloppy handling of fridge doors really annoyed me. 'This is my night's sleep that's wasted!' I'd think, and get really upset. And the milk flow was going down to adjust to the demand Tuffel actually made on the breast. There is only so much a woman can pump at night. Even while watching *Horrible Histories*. Sleep is still more appealing.

I doubted I'd make my record-breaking goal of 50 litres and wondered if I could slow things down and give up on the project, so I started preparing my positively framed 'press statement' about it. There is the 'press statement' and there is what's really going on. When what's really going on is too complex or painful to say, I revert to a socially acceptable press statement. I came up with this when I lived in Berlin and went to the University of Performing Arts. Saying "I study musical theatre" was a great press statement answer to "What are you doing these days?". The full and truthful answer I'd give to those who were close enough was more along the lines of: "I'm exploring myself and the world of music, spirituality and the borders of insanity. I don't know where this is going, I feel I'm going mad at times and there is something deeply unexpressed and painful I'm trying to figure out. I've had some pretty intense experiences with myself that don't sound normal nor mentally stable and I'm determined to find answers and happiness by exploring the truth about life." And because that's way too much for most to swallow or relate to, I've learned to create these 'press statements'.

My ambition to deliver a record-breaking amount of milk was disproportionally important to me, and my failure was causing me grief. "Who cares, babe? You're doing amazing!" was Thomas' more practical and clear approach. *I* cared. A lot. In a world where you can't control much, the little things you think you can sometimes carry more weight than is rational. It's a way of coping, some would say. It's just a way to make oneself feel in control. I get that. So my way of being in charge was to set a goal and feel I can still achieve something. Another way I made myself feel I was in charge was by neatly folding my clothes in my cupboard. I might not be able to control the health and life of my son, but I can control the creases of my clothes in the cupboard. So I do. Sometimes. When I can be arsed.

Meanwhile, in hospital, Tuffel likes ripping out his nasal tube. He might be a gentle soul, the type who looks at a rose in wonder, but he's certainly not gentle with a tube in his nose. I'd say it's the nurses' job to ensure the tube stays in by plastering it properly. Hearing a nurse say "I'd better fix that soon" fills me with dread – it means it will be out by the time they're back. The newer nurses go through that experience at least once. Talk about learning the hard way – they were learning and Tuffel was getting it the hard way. Inserting the tube is just harsh. Imagine someone shoving a phone cable through your nostril, throat and through your stomach, poking around until they'd think they made it to the bowel. X-ray, check. Wrong place, let's go again. X-ray, check. Each tube-fixing could take one to three days. It was ongoing. Tuffel had more X-rays than you and me put together.

I hear X-rays aren't good for you, but they are the best we can do for my son right now. They are certainly useful for checking if that tube is finally in the right place. I can't really keep up with all the things that aren't good for you, so I surrender. If you can't beat them, join them. At some point they started inserting the tubes under continuous radiation, which was a much calmer procedure, as the radiologist would see where he/she was going at any point. It meant 200 or so X-rays per session rather than two to eight, but it meant so much less distress, too. While this is going on, I get to wear these incredible designer lead skirts and vests. Talk about a silver lining – this one is made of real lead! If you wear those you don't need to worry about your figure. I was never a fan of heavy metal, but I appreciate the protective wear a lot. The best feature is the Velcro fasteners: taking this off not only makes me feel light as a feather – shedding a fair few pounds in a few seconds – it also has striptease quality to it only I seem to get. Well, the staff in the room get a laugh when I strut my stuff, musical-theatre style. You've got to have fun when you can.

In one of these now regular radiology sessions, a strange white line appeared on screen. Turns out a tube ending had broken off and got stuck in his stomach. Tube endings don't just break off. I tried to tear one – I couldn't. It's a complete mystery how it happened, but there it was. Four centimetres of plastic tubing.

So our favourite surgeon, Miss Agrawal, our team of consultants, Thomas and I decided to change the plumbing system and get a gastrostomy for Tuffel – this would involve a tube being inserted into the stomach, with a second one going into the bowel through the tummy tube.

It's the operation we had prevented a few months ago, but back then, the nasal solution was working splendidly. Back then we weren't regular customers at the radiologist's basement procedure rooms. As confident as I was getting at my lead costume dress up and striptease routine, we knew we couldn't go on like this. When inserting the new permanent stomach access (gastrostomy) they could remove that bit of plastic, too. It was stuck and couldn't come out any other way. Hospital life involves frequent changes of scenarios. One must remain flexible to adjust, cope and find the best solutions at any given time. I suppose this can be said for all of life.

We had to secure a date with our surgeon, who's always busy, and the radiologists. And make sure a theatre was available too, and hope that no emergency bumped us off the list. When I say 'we', I mean the medical team, but Thomas and I also wanted to be around. Thomas had some important meetings coming up and wanted to make sure he could be there on the big day. The doctors tried to hunt our surgeon down, to no avail. I found her. Where? At my second home, the Neonatal Unit. Apparently I'm not the only one who likes to hang out there.

Dr Meena Agrawal is one of UK's top 10 paediatric surgeons. A dignified lady, she is smaller than me (I like when I meet someone smaller than me as it doesn't happen all that often). Miss Agrawal, also known as Miss A to those less confident in pronouncing her last name, looks like the wise woman of the tribe. I could sit and listen to her for hours. I can't because she's way too busy saving lives. She fills me with such a sense of awe and desire to get the best out of myself. She used to climb mountains and she works for four different hospitals rescuing babies with her surgical magic – what an honour to have her care for us.

This time around Thomas and I both accompanied Tuffel to theatre and sent him off to sleep. I tried to stop the worrying thoughts running through my mind as I saw my son with a gas mask over his face.

Miss A asked me with a glimmer in her eye: so, how's the milk donation going? "I'm at 40 litres," I said, slightly deflated, getting ready to bring some kind of reasoning why I wouldn't achieve my goal. But she couldn't care less about that. "This woman ought to be applauded for what she does! Did you hear that? That's incredible!" she announced to the room. My face was now beaming. Acknowledgment of that kind does something very powerful to me. And in that moment I knew I wasn't going to give up.

I wanted to really give my best and report back. It was, after all, for a good cause. However, I was going to change my approach. The goal itself became less important and the 'how I get there' more important. I could be good to others and good to myself. I didn't have to beat myself or others up over every bottle.

Later that day, I met Lindsey, another mum, who was waiting for her little one to get a pea taken out of his lungs. As she recalled the moment Franklin was gassed to a slumber, tears were brought to my eyes, too. It always brings it home to me when someone else goes through the same experience. We had a beautiful moment bonding in our pain. I'm so glad our kids are much better with anaesthetics than us big babies. And at the same time these events have immense bonding potential. Pain shared is pain halved they say in German. Or, as Thomas puts it: "It's nice how you make new friends over a crying session."

During his operation, a small camera was slid down Tuffel's throat. A hole was drilled into the stomach. Tube #1 inserted. Tube #2 inserted into tube #1 and advanced under constant X-ray to the bowel. Surgical fishing line thrown in to catch the old forgotten tube bit that was happily rotting in the bowel pouch. We had signed the document to allow an 'open procedure' to take place should this not work out. They would have to cut the belly open to access the stomach and it would be a bigger operation. Luckily, the 'fishing' worked just fine and the whole thing could be done in a keyhole surgery sort of way. No open procedure necessary after all. Little Tuffmeister was stable and snoozing. We were so relieved to have him back in our arms after one and a half hours.

We didn't, however, expect the level of screaming we faced the next couple of days. Thank God for painkillers. Thomas kept asking if we made the right decision. It's easy to doubt oneself when confronted with a child in pain. We just want him to feel good! I'd take his pain for him if I could. It's not my choice. We have to live with the consequences of our actions and we allowed this to happen in good faith that it will be the best for Tuffel. Patience and self-kindness were needed. A few days later, when Tuffel could feed again and the soreness subsided, the situation became quite clear: this is amazing. Tuffel's face is now free from tubes. No more itching or allergic reaction to the plasters. No more pulling. The redness has healed up. For the first time in five months we can see his face fully. The chubby cheeks! With his waste bags now at waist level (the stoma bag and the drainage bag), we tuck them into his clothes and carry him around like a normal baby. Sure, if you take his clothes off you will see the complex logistics going on that support this miracle. But with clothes, you just can't tell. I'm so excited. My overwhelming desire to be 'normal' is being satisfied to a superficial degree, which means so much more than expected.

On an outing to the dentist, the receptionist exclaimed: "Oh, such a cute baby! Look at him, not a care in the world!" Wow – we must really look normal to her. How incredible. But wait a minute. Not a care? He hasn't had his arm in a shirt sleeve until a week ago, has cuddled his mother in a bed twice so far, and he lives on machines! He was told he can't survive, lives without a vital organ in a state of uncertainty and has huge scars on his body. And that's only the beginning. How dare you be so ignorant? What? What would you know?

I didn't say any of that, of course. These kind of thoughts offer themselves up so readily and in bulk. I know where they lead, the tightness they trigger in my tummy, the weight they put on my mood. I chose not to think them through. I stopped at "If only you knew – he's been through a lot". Enough. I don't have to go there.

I chose to smile and not to speak. Isn't it nice she can see the beauty and wholeness in him? That she perceives us as just another mum and baby walking in? Isn't that what I wanted? Reflecting on her words now, I agree: he doesn't have a worry to hold on to. He doesn't know the concept of worry. That's adult stuff. So, again, I get to learn from my little man. Because I, too, do not need to hold on to worries. They pass. I don't need to hold on to the cares in the world. Life is good when we are taking it one cheeky smile at a time.

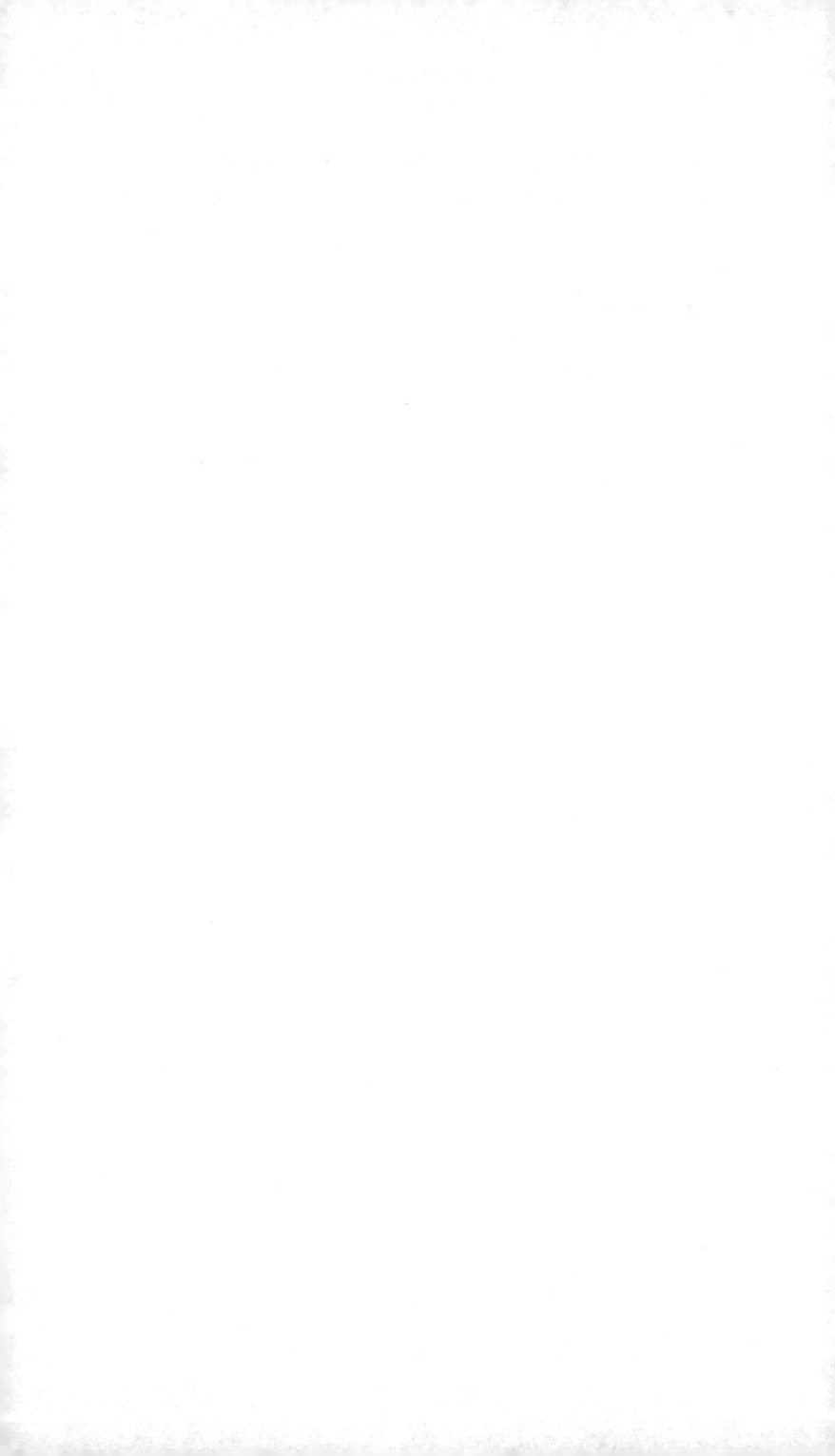

CHAPTER 13:

Life at Evelina Children's Hospital

(6 MONTHS)

It took time to get used to life at the Evelina Children's Hospital. When Tuffel contracted a virus, he was sent into isolation. At first that was my idea of a nightmare because the thought my six-month old baby lying in a room on his own made me cringe. Yes, six months. Half a crazy year.

But, as it turns out, Mr T is really good on his own, chatting away and engaging in heated discussions with Sophie the Giraffe (that ubiquitous rubber teething toy that squeaks with every bite and squeeze). I don't know what she did to him and given that her head is mainly in his mouth, I do think she's really the one who has more reason to complain, but she just grins and bears it. He can certainly get into a huff – it sounds like he's really telling her off – followed by a much-needed cooling down period sucking that thumb.

He is good at charming the nurses, and Sheryl in particular did a fab job of loving him back. He got a routine and a day plan. No longer will he accept my milk in a bottle. He would rather wait till I come in. Tuffel believes in boobs. He wants them on demand. Thomas finds it unfair – nobody finds it cute when he has the same request.

The hospital's play specialist or physios come in the morning and the nurses get their cuddles in before I take over. At first I would go back to my friends in the Neonatal Unit every time we had the chance, but since we contracted a viral infection, we have been staying clear. I don't want to cause harm to the little premature babies. Instead, I take the bus home in the day, with my baby in the buggy. Just like any normal mum, squeezing onto a London bus coughing and sneezing. In the evening, Thomas drives us back. We have a car now, which makes our life a lot easier. My mummy-friend Caroline from my NCT group moved to Hong Kong and gave us her hers. And to make sure it's okay, she had it serviced first, too. How generous is that? I will never cease to be amazed by how wonderful people can be and how unexpectedly good things can happen.

As is the case so often in life, what we think of as bad can turn out to be quite good, if we choose to see the good in it. The isolation cubicle, for example, was a blessing in disguise: it turned out to be a private room with en suite bathroom. Space to spread out the stuff we've accumulated. When I close the door, I don't hear other patients' machines beeping anymore. I can lie on the plastic couch and feed, whereas the new rule in the bay forbids us to take the bed down in the daytime. Rules in hospitals can be quite random. Some can be broken, some can't. The bed-down rule? No chance. The rule that you can't use the 'helter skelter' slide in the play area if you're over 4ft tall? Well… try and stop me.

Did I mention that I asked for some more contrast studies to be done of Tuffel's intestine? I wanted to see how much it had grown. Dr Agrawal looked me straight in the eyes: "You know it's not possible for it to grow. You are asking for a miracle!" I held her gaze. "Yes, I am." We locked eyes. And she ordered the studies. "I suppose there is no real harm," she said. After two weeks, the consultants told me that though the bowel had grown, it was only proportionally to his body and therefore of no further significance. Sorry.

The month went past, the flu symptoms subsided and the time came for our final transfer to King's Hospital.

At King's, we'd get our final training in administering the artificial nutrition (TPN) so that we could go home. In the NHS, you have to be a trained nurse, get IV training on top and then you're allowed to learn to handle TPN, which requires extra training and certification. Because infection must be avoided at all costs, we were trained in the principles of aseptic technique and working in a sterile environment. The nurses use what is known as ANTT. Aseptic Non-Touch Technique. It means you learn not to touch any of the key parts of equipment involved. We are being trained in a sterile way, so not only do we not touch, we wear sterile gloves and work with sterile fields to add another layer of protection. I call it OTT ANTT (Over-the-Top Aseptic Non-Touch Technique). It makes me proud to be able to pronounce it and the nurses have a laugh with us.

There is a whole lot to organise, as all the ancillaries of the artificial nutrition will have to be ordered to our house on a regular basis. We need to boil down what they are specifically and how many we'll need each month. You'd think that's already written down somewhere as a standardised process, but everything needs to be adapted to our needs. We use a variety of dressings and bags that not everyone would use because our situation is unique. I hold on to every piece of equipment I like, jot down the reference number and complicated name and hand it over to the nutrition nurse who is compiling the big order.

I know that they won't have the same things at King's that that they have at St Thomas'/Evelina, so I have to make sure I pack supplies from here and take them there. Enough to use and to show the staff so they can order them in for us. Apart from about 40 different items we'll need, we also need help. It's going to be a different life doing all the care that four nurses did, by myself: nobody wants me to break down in the middle of it.

First, I went back to the Neonatal Unit (that's St. Thomas') to give out my thank you cards and celebrate in style with my dear friends and fellow neonatal survivors, Claire and Elaine, whose company had meant the world to us over the last six months. Claire had made a cappuccino cake and even brought her little Casper out to the parents' room. With his oxygen canister. Casper is a week older than Tuffel. After struggling with his breathing for six months, he was waiting to have a tracheostomy (a hole in the throat with a whistle-like construction held by a sort of Elizabethan collar that helps you breathe). Elaine's girl had been born at 23 weeks – a full-term pregnancy is 37-39 weeks. Her oxygen levels had been going up and down; many times we feared for her life. She had never left her little cot. So this was truly an exciting event! A very exclusive tea gathering in the parents' room. It's just outside the ward, so if anything were to happen, the nurses are 10 seconds away. It was quite emotional and the opposite of relaxed, with everyone on high alert, but life is what it is and we were having a really special moment. With some pretty amazing cake. It was a bit like a mums' outing at

Starbucks. We had buggies and baby talk. Just exchange the coffee machine with suctioning devices and the cafe atmosphere for hospital-blue walls and you're there.

It's hard to believe we are really going to our last hospital stop before home, but it's real: our bouncing chair, pictures, books and toys packed, we were transferred (or rather, sent off in a minicab) to King's. Having been there several times during the transplant assessment, it felt more like a homecoming. The nurses were excited to see us and we felt welcomed at once. We were finally with the consultants who understand short gut (better) and how to manage his cares properly. Goodbye boring discussions with paediatricians new to the case. No more explaining that, yes, we are using medical devices in the opposite way to what they're usually employed for.

Having been nicely prepped by the St Thomas' crew, we started our official training. If you'd have told me that one day I'd be taking bloods, wearing sterile gloves and a mask, doing an IV nurse's job for my child, I'd have said 'Yeah, right'. I would have laughed at you while doing a headstand.

So, as much as we can plan what we'll do when we grow up, I've come to realise that real 'growing up' is about showing grace when it comes to the unplanned. Doing what needs to be done with a smile *and* nurturing our essential connection to our dreams and what we love.

Thomas and I both know how to do the aseptic procedures: we draw blood and handle syringes like you see in the movies. I change the dressings of Tuffel's lines – that's something the doctors do at the Neonatal Unit – oh, it's a whole new skill set. If I was still acting, it would so go on my CV under 'other skills', next to rollerskating (basic level) and my clean driving licence (none of their business how many stains I got on that paper). All I need now is the nursing uniform. Although I'll probably opt for the one from Ann Summers as they fit much better – who said home life had to be boring?

Thomas finally had his last test regarding his intestines. This involved swallowing a camera pill, which takes 100,000 pictures on its journey to the other end of his bowel. Thank God we don't have to fish it out and develop the film! The images are transmitted via radio signal to a device. How intrusive can a camera get? Let's call it the Pooperazzi Pill. I hope we won't get the results from the front pages of a magazine – if we did, it certainly wouldn't be *OK!* It could be *Readers Digest* or *Runner's World*. Okay, you might not have laughed, but I can assure you the gastroenterology endoscopy nurse did.

And since London is currently in the midst of Olympics fever, I think it's worth mentioning that I proudly beat the record for milk donation to the Neonatal Unit at St Thomas' Hospital, London, GB, which was 50 litres, after all. That's a lot of milk coming from one set of boobies. The milk bank nurses even laughed off my ambition: "You and your milk record." They even said once: "You can't keep bringing your milk here". I think that nurse must have had a bad night's sleep. She wouldn't really want to deny the life-saving donation. She was probably the one who had to count the milk and sterilise it. I'm too proud to get annoyed. I think they'd better cut out that cardboard gold star. I made 60 litres of bottled love. Six zero! When are they adding breast milk pumping to the list of Olympic sports anyway? I promise you the seats wouldn't be empty!

But most importantly, *Tuffel is coming home* – we have a date. It's Tuesday, July 13!

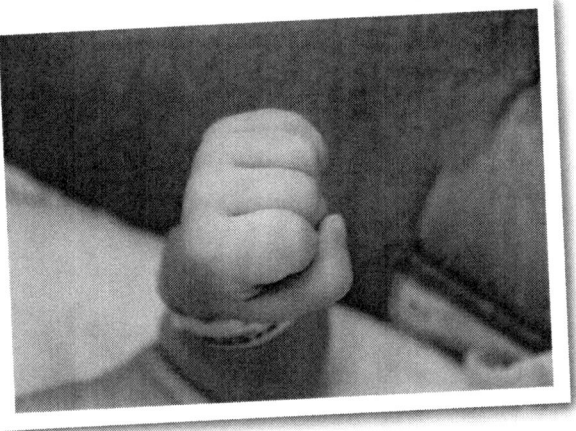

CHAPTER 14

There is no place like... Can I please go now?

(7 MONTHS)

Well, we thought Tuffel's homecoming would be on the 13th of July. Make that the 2nd of August – it didn't quite happen as planned...

We were meant to be at King's for two weeks to learn about aseptic technique and the pumps that will be part of Tuffel's home routine. Tuffel is now being fed his sterile 'space food' (TPN) straight into his bloodstream over 12 hours each night. That means he's hooked up to a pump and a bag that streams all the nutrients, fats and liquids directly into his blood. No need to digest and absorb. He's off the hook in the daytime. We've come such a long way from the days when he was on a 24/7 feeding stream!

Because we are dealing with a line ending at the top right heart chamber, all handlings of that line need to be aseptic (without the presence of bacteria), hence all the extensive training in OTT ANTT. The last task was to learn how to set the pumps and understand the various alarms. Followed by events to roll your eyes at: Lambeth Council had forgotten to assign the home care contract to a company before our care nurse went on holiday, so the process got delayed by 10 days. Our training itself was delayed for a week because of another person's annual leave. Add another week.

It seemed to be a confusing and mind-boggling task to get all the supplies together and ordered. Caroline was putting her heart and soul into getting us home, running around sorting out supplies, organizing rooms for training, she was instructing us and managing everyone involved. She had to convince the community nurses that we are ok using nasal gastric tubes for his recycling even though they are made to be used through he nose not through the tummy. The community nurse didn't want to know. "The product specifies the way it should be used. We will not supply it for any other use as it's against the regulations". But what we do is new and doesn't have products to support it so we use what works. This works. Yes it's safe. As far as we know and that's all we'll ever know!

Caroline couldn't have been more approachable and personable. Having genuinely caring people on the team makes all the difference. Even when we got frustrated about the delays, we knew we were cared for.

We have an Excel sheet full of ancillaries to be ordered each item has a name a long reference number and some code. Get one thing wrong and it won't show up in the system. The TPN has to be prescribed via the pharmacists and deliveries need to be established. About one family a year is sent home on TPN from King's Hospital, eight so far in total. As a result, there is no routine when it comes to this process. There are huge files with rules to be adhered to and busy people trying to make them work. The numbers of Home PN patients (that's what Tuffel will be) are rising, but it's so new that they don't even have a proper register of how many families live with Home PN! PN stands for Parenteral Nutrition. Some people have a little to top up their normal eating when they can't digest enough food due to a short gut or a disease. Tuffel is fully dependent on it so in his case it's TPN – Total Parenteral Nutrition. That's where he takes ALL his nutrients from. Tuffel's initials are saved in the national register being created at the moment. Since artificial nutrition is now working better – even for long-term patients – we will see a rise in people plugged into parenteral feeding.

I had been house hunting like crazy. I'd seen most of Crystal Palace and Sydenham before Thomas remembered that thanks to an old skiing injury, a hilly neighbourhood would not be suitable for his knees – especially in winter.

But I just couldn't find anything that Thomas and I could agree on, and when we did it was outside the budget. Or too far from public transport. In the meantime, house prices kept rising along with our frustration and tension. I'm going to introduce a new word for the state we experienced more often than anyone would want: frustension. I remember reporting back to Doctor Hind that I just couldn't find what we wanted and we couldn't afford to stay in our area. "We'll have to get social services involved then; "they will find you a place." My mouth ran dry. Frustension turned into shock. I didn't want to be rude, but was he really referring to a council flat? I appreciate help but I really don't see myself living in a council flat. No offence, but we have aspirations. Maybe we're a bit spoilt, but we like it pretty. Plus, we are doing way too well to accept that sort of help. We were just being priced out of our area. I felt a little shame to say it, but then again we didn't want to spend half a million on a small two bedroom flat even if we did have the money. I've seen two bedroom terraced houses around the corner for 800k. No swimming pool, no golden taps. But I think they throw in some drafty windows instead. And a fireplace you're not allowed to use, but it looks cosy. No thank you! It took me courage and calm to decline the offer for help. I didn't want to sound more arrogant than I am. "Are you sure we can't fit the stuff into our flat in the meantime? We'll keep searching, of course". And so the Neonatal Outreach Team came to visit our flat and suggested we move our bed from the bedroom to the living room to make space for the equipment in the bedroom. The living room of 4m x 4m had a desk, bookshelves, the piano, Tuffel's new changing station and chest of drawers and a couch in it. Thomas works from there, too. But hey, who needs furniture when you have a double bed?

How many boxes of equipment were we actually talking about? At first we were told it was a six month supply. Then it was maybe three months. Why don't people just say "we don't know" and find out? A phone call to Bupa months later had clarified that we were actually talking about a one month supply of ancillaries. TPN goes into a big fridge and would be delivered weekly. So how many boxes would that be? We would only find out on the day of delivery. Which was the day before Tuffel's discharge. So we ran with it. We'd manage somehow. Mission impossible? Not really. Mission "are you crazy?" – that has my name on it. Bring it on. We'd done much bigger things in the last eight months. At least we had an approximate fridge measurement and the space under our staircase looked like it might take it. Goodbye, shoe shelf.

When I came home on supply delivery day I burst out laughing. Was that what all the fuss had been about?

Seriously? The pressure to find a new house for 10 moving boxes? Sure, they would have to find a more accessible space than being piled on top of each other in the hallway leaving very little room to manoeuvre, but I had heard of a new invention we could make use of. It's called a shelf.

So, finally, the big day came and at the discharge planning meeting, a Bupa nurse showed us how to use the pump. It looked so easy! The home pumps are nothing like the clumsy, constantly beeping monstrosities we endured in Neonatal. We were eager to practise using it. I could hear Thomas' breathing restrict slightly when he tried it, and I could feel myself being rather short-fused when it was my turn. We look calm and we do well, but it's quite daunting to think about the importance of getting it right.

Our goal is to prevent line infections. They are the biggest obstacles. Infections are nasty and they can cause veins to close down as well as risk little T's life if not caught early. As there are only four entry points for TPN into the body, it's crucial we keep the line as long as possible. The other big obstacle is liver damage. TPN can be hard on the liver and has destroyed some in the past. Tuffel has already recovered from TPN-induced jaundice, that clever little boy. His liver is working beautifully for now.

I try not to think about all this when I'm doing it. To be honest, it's only when I begin to write it all down that I can evaluate where the tension draws from. It's best to not think about the consequences when I engage in Tuffel's cares. I just do what needs to be done: spike the bag, draw up my saline, get the air out of the line when priming. That's all. One crucial step at a time. It's not the end of the world if we make a mistake; we just need to realise what we did in order to make the right choices with our adjustments. This can involve a simple glove change to discarding the bag of TPN entirely. A hundred pounds worth of dinner. If the connecting element has touched something, it has to go. There is no room for covering up, muddling through or getting away with errors.

I admire Thomas, who constantly questions the processes and the logic behind them. It's easy to get institutionalised – accept what has been said by someone whom we assume knows better. Thomas will only accept what he understands. We changed a few processes because we prefer them to make sense to us. Being new to the game meant we brought a different awareness with us, which had the nurses stop in their tracks and rethink their work, too. The ones happy to learn loved us for it; others, not so much.

The Rays of Sunshine children's ward at King's is outstanding. The respect and support we got from our nurses was incredible. Again, I felt we had a home, a community we belonged to. Having spent most of my working life as a solo artist and solopreneur, it has been a tremendously enriching experience to be part of a team in this way.

So we knew how to set things up, we had the pump, everything was ready to go. The original idea was that we'd room in for a few nights, taking over all the cares, but still be in reach of help if need be. But reality had a different plan. Hospitals draw on charities like Ronald McDonald House to provide accommodation for the families of long-term patients. Yes it's *that* McDonald, whom you either love or hate. Also, the Samaritans have some rooms they lend to King's.

Unfortunately, when we needed it, there was no flat available for us, so I was going to have to do this solo. And instead of being in a room with Tuffel, we were relocated to the nursery. Into the smallest bed space of the ward, with three other babies in the room. Babies who were very unwell. I did get upset about it, but can you really stay angry in a ward where children are awaiting their third liver transplant or suffering from undiagnosed intestinal failure? I cannot really feel sorry for myself for long when I see little Mohammed (name has been changed) being wheeled up and down the corridor, yellow eyes poking out of his dark skin. The dark skin is genetic; the yellow eyes are from liver disease. Time is ticking as he waits for an organ. Neema (name changed for privacy) isn't growing. She's been here for months on end. Her new liver works fine, but she's still not growing. She walks to the playroom with her drip stand, and the nurses will do her cares while she's on the Nintendo Wii or recites her favourite book, which she now knows by heart.

I enjoy the playroom, which is a lovely meeting place for parents and kids. We do some arts and crafts, and Tuffy loves watching the fish in the aquarium and making new friends. Everyone loves seeing Tuff. His smiles are infectious. Infectious is maybe a little inappropriate to say in a transplant ward where we don't like infection but you know… we wash our hands all the time. Still, his good mood is contagious.

So, time for me to spend a night with Tuffel and the new pump, make sure it all works and then go home! I was in excellent spirits. Setting up was challenging because the order in which we set up and administer the TPN is different from the hospital pumps on which we had been trained. And in a world where one unsterile touch means you need to start again or throw away the whole bag, it's a big deal.

I didn't really expect to sleep much. Between alarms and cries, I finally found some rest. Until I hear an alarm that I wasn't used to – not to worry, the nurse will sort it out in the next five minutes. I hope. Beep Beep Beep Beep. Or is that my alarm? 'Oh no, wait,' says my brain, you have to sort this out – that's why you're here. Of course. I snapped out of my daze, adrenaline rushing through my body. What's that about? The pump says 'battery near end'. But it's in the charger. The plug was on, the cable is in, the battery was fully charged. We had been told it can run for two days or so. Beep Beep Beep. I am waking up the whole hospital. Pushing all sorts of buttons. Nothing happens. The nurse comes in but nobody knows this pump. I can't stop it. Beep Beep Beep. It's going to wake up all of London. I rush out to call the emergency hotline while the nurse is trying to fiddle with the pump. The Bupa representative doesn't know what to do except send me a new pump within three hours. Tuffel needs his food. Now. A sudden stop is really unhealthy for the blood sugar. We try to swap back to the hospital pumps but they use different attachments (administration sets) – in other words, it's not possible – so we have to put him onto a drip with a dextrose solution. Tuffel wakes up from all the rushing around him, startled.

He must have felt the stress –he started coughing. Then throwing up. Then I notice the bed is completely wet. His nappy stinks – it's just pee, but it's everywhere. The nappy weighs almost half a kilo. I'm so confused. Beep Beep and then silence. The pump just dies.

This is bad. If we'd been home, we would have been blue-lighted into the nearest hospital. My stress levels are somewhere near the top of the roof. You can't tell; I act rather calm. But inside I'm shaking. I pick him up, my golden boy, the nurse changes the sheet. How on earth am I going to do this at home? I change his nappy, his clothes. We put him on the drip, the doctor prescribes a sugar bolus (a dose of sugar solution infused intravenously). Urine, vomit, dangerously low blood sugar levels, syringes, stool, doctors, chaos. What's next? What does it mean? I can't take him home like this! And indeed, he needs to recover, we need a new pump and we need to start over again. Our confidence is shaken. Will we be stranded with sleepless nights and high dramas? Once we are out of the system, will they still care? Would it not be better to bring him back at night to be on the safe side? We want our boy home, but at what cost?

Bupa sent us two new pumps. Thomas and I test them with bags of saline (salt water). And somehow they don't really work so well. The filter doesn't take the air out, alarms keep going off. I send one back and receive another one. It's a week later and I am ready to start again. We hook him up and alarms we were told did not exist go off. What the heck now? I couldn't figure it out. I call the hotline. The nurse on the other end says she doesn't know this pump. She can only give me generic advice. At 4p per minute that may be a good deal if I ever needed generic advice. If you are ever in need of some generic advice in the middle of the night, try 0845 757 3100.

I didn't need generic advice. I needed help with *this* freaking pump. I want to take my boy home and still sleep at night. We lost our trust in the home pumps.

We researched pumps and found that the Rythmic model is popular. Even though the musician in me notices the spelling mistake: there should be an H after the R. I hope that this tiny device will give us what we need. As Gloria Estefan sings: 'The rhythm is going to get you, the rhythm is going to get you – tonight'. Our hospital go-to person is fine with it, but Bupa needs the council to approve the funds. An extra £12-£15,000. Each pump costs around £3k and we need two pumps, plus backup. Needless to say, things got stuck again in the channels of communication. In times of recession, is this going too far? We grew incredibly frustrated and tense.

Not only because we'd been looking forward to going home for a long time and were delayed by three weeks at this point, but because I'd booked a holiday. Yes. Because once we are placed on the transplant list, we'd have to remain within one hour from the hospital at all times. This could be for the next months or years, we couldn't know. I thought it would be a good idea to take Tuffel to France for a week, have some quality time at the Villa Westenholz (that's what I call Thomas' family's holiday home). Everyone had been in favour of the idea – even though it would be a huge effort logistically, the consensus was: You gotta live. And I love to live.

But it all seemed to fall apart at the seams. No pumps, low blood sugar levels in the mornings, found during random checks – and infrequent vomits. Things just kept dragging on and on. In between we were busy choosing care package providers, meeting the hospice outreach team and organising simple things, like a German passport. This is where my organisational skills came in very handy. Using categorised lists to keep track of it all. Chasing the providers, the council, getting an emergency appointment at the embassy. Have you ever communicated with German bureaucrats? You usually need three to six months to get an appointment to apply for a passport. I got one in a week – a small victory.

My other achievement was to introduce the name Tuffel to the German name register. In Germany you can't just name your children Apple Blossom or Peach or Soda Pop, as people do over here. You must name a child by a name that exists and clarifies the gender. Oh, the discussions we could have had. As Tuffel was born in London, he was registered at Lambeth Town Hall under the name of Tuffel and the German Embassy will not argue with a birth certificate. They are Germans, after all, and we value official documents – we don't argue with those. If you are German and would like to name your next child Tuffel, you can officially do so. There is a German Tuffel, and you can prove it. It is now an official name! Get out your Weissbeer and Bratwurst to celebrate with me.

During those weeks I barely spoke to anyone in my family. Nor my friends. There was just too much going on and during the minutes I did have free; I just needed the silence. Plus, repeating the details of the ordeals we'd been through was too tedious. What you are reading here, I promise, is only the outline of what was going on.

Third time lucky, I spent another night at the hospital with our shiny new Rythmic pump and my Tuffmeister. By now, I knew that I had to change his diapers throughout the night. Tuffel sleeps through the night – it's every new mother's dream. But because he gets all his fluid intake during that time, he wees like a native Bavarian at the Oktoberfest. So up I get. And as for the vomiting, well, I suppose he's just behaving like an American teenager visiting the Oktoberfest.

Our consultant is calm about it. After all, it's not beer but Tuffel's anatomy that's causing this. But then again, he doesn't have to change the sheets and fight with a washer/dryer that is fickle about which clothes it likes to wash and which ones it likes to get stuck on program 14 (open door; get surprised by very wet clothes).

I'm happy to report that the Rythmic has indeed gotten me and all went well. Hurrah. It was time to pack up. What a surreal day. One last bath and dressing change. Carrying the green 'patient's property' bags to the car. Collecting Tuffel after his last cuddles with his favourite nurses. Actually saying goodbye.

This was not another transfer. This was a discharge. I was in a state of disbelief until I had the letter confirming it in my hand. We were going home. Home to our one bedroom flat. I haven't found a bigger one yet. We'll just have to fit all his stuff in somewhere. We don't need access to the garden, do we?

It's been seven months. We were finally taking our little boy into our care. From here on he would sleep in his own little cot. No more white hospital sheets. Get out the cute baby bedding with pictures of cars and buses! No more dragging clean clothes into hospital and dirty ones home. Goodbye schlepping nappies around on public transport, hello pine chest of drawers with changing station! No more knocking before entering the medicine storage room to get my supplies, hello tons of boxes overcrowding our tiny hallway! No more getting annoyed at the porters for bringing up the TPN late and hello extra-large fridge under our staircase! No more running to the station to catch a train to pick up the baby and hello waking up with my baby in the bedroom at 6:15am.

Wow. We are going to be parents.

We have contact numbers and equipment flowcharts and who-does-what-lists and a fit-for-travel letter. We have a car full of stuff and, oh my word, now we have our little miracle boy.

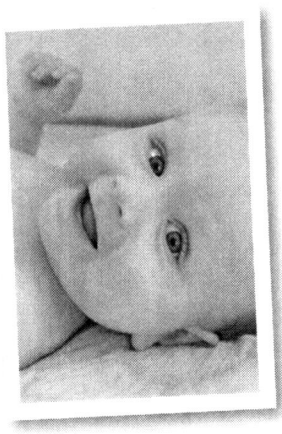

CHAPTER 15

Holiday... Celebrate!

(8 MONTHS)

He's home. Looking at little Wonderboy in the morning, beaming at us first thing, is fantastic. It trumps the old routine of getting up and ready, reminding myself to clean the breakfast bowls because they don't clean themselves, grabbing the batch of clean clothes, running to catch a train, waiting, riding, up the steps, beep the Oyster card, getting to hospital, through the building, the long corridors, heading to the third floor – "Good morning everyone!" – hand washing, hand sanitising, "How are you?". And, finally, "Helloooo Tuffel!" It beats it a million times for sure. All that is OVER.

"Eah grrr ssst cht kr," says our little man, and up I get, peeling myself out of the bed. And there he is: wet, stinky nappy and big smile. The pumps are buzzing – four more minutes till we need to disconnect. Better wake up and create a sterile field. Thomas is doing his silly dance. It's a good day. My eyes are heavy. I've been up during the night and I sleep lightly. With every sound he makes, I am up to check on him. He sometimes coughs and vomits at night, which sounds dramatic, so the adrenaline kicks in as I twist his little body around to make it easier. The lines are always in the way. I have to keep calm, they mustn't get pulled. Never mind. He goes back to sleep minutes later. And I'm too tired to stay up for long. It's great having him home. He's our little boy. Finally.

I suppose a 'welcome home Tuffel' party would be appropriate. But staying home isn't exactly what Thomas and I have in mind…

As Thomas was in need of a 'man trip', he had booked himself a sailing course a while back. I remember that a long time ago, I was the one who proclaimed that you can live your dream, even with a child. But then came life. Instead of going to the Edinburgh Festival, I went to the Evelina Children's Hospital; instead of soaking up the sun, we ended up in the Rays of Sunshine ward… but still. I think Thomas should still enjoy a little adventure – it's something he's longed for.

But what about my dreams? Well, I love France and relaxing at the Villa Westenholz. And where there is a wish, there might just be a way to fulfil it. I had the tickets booked, I just needed all the extra bits and pieces to get sorted – including feeling comfortable enough with the equipment to unleash myself into the wilderness of Central Europe. With all the pump disasters and delays, I had exactly 10 days to accomplish it all before take-off.

Planning a holiday with a bowel-less baby is a bit like counting the hair on your legs – it just never seems to end, and seems like it's going nowhere. But this was also an opportunity to revive some skills I'd learned in a former life when I worked as a corporate events producer and later coordinator in the licensing industry. Organising what seems impossible in a short amount of time? Let's do it! The 40 different medical items we need had to be packed in various quantities. Plus there was travel insurance, the correct letters from the hospital, the special delivery of

TPN to the airport, and a suitable fridge at the destination to be arranged – just to name a few of the tasks on my to-do list. Packing the 'normal' baby things? That was the last on my list. It can be daunting to a new mum, so here is my tip for everyone packing for their first holiday with a baby and this is how I did it: open closet, take out stuff, close closet. Done.

I suppose it was a very ambitious undertaking to go on an overseas holiday with all of Tuffel's medical stuff. I now know that many families with members on TPN don't leave the comfort of their own home, let alone their country. The second ambitious undertaking? Doing it on my own. Thomas was going to enjoy his sailing and I was going to enjoy France.

On that note, I have to give a big thank you to PINNT, the association for people in need of artificial nutrition (yes, there is a support group after all). Their holiday guide and tips were not only encouraging but very practical and saved me days of work. It's invaluable to have the support of people in similar situations.

I had three suitcases, a buggy, a car seat, the rucksack with the pumps, two large boxes of TPN at 12.5kg each, my handbag and the baby. It took two trolleys to carry it all, plus the buggy, which, admittedly, was a little hard to push on my own. When I asked for help at the disability help point, I got told off. "You don't want wheelchair assistance?" No, I don't. But someone to help with my stuff please. "This is only for wheelchair assistance!"

When systems fail, it's always good to remember that people can be amazing. I got help from fellow travellers. I should have counted the looks I got for schlepping my stuff around with a varying cast of helpers. Asking for help really goes a long way. As does being kind. Just as the check-in assistant understood my situation, the supervisor – "I *am* the supervisor" – had to butt in and contact customer service to find out if I could indeed transport all my gear. I could feel my inner kettle starting to boil my blood into English Breakfast. Then I realised he was just a busy man trying to do a good job. Before he could give me the verdict I asked him for his name. "Thank you for helping me today, Dimitri. I understand it's busy and you are understaffed. I appreciate you are taking the time to accommodate my needs." Mr I-*am*-the-supervisor became Mr Super: he arranged for people to help me carry the bags, and made sure I wouldn't get charged for all the extra equipment on the way back. Brilliant.

On the plane, Tuffel showed off his comprehension skills: reaching for the laminated information card as instructed by the bored-looking stewardess, he looked at it with great concentration. Well, I suppose it was the first time he was instructed about emergency exits and slides we would hopefully never need to use. I'm glad he studied it so well. My seat neighbour was rather impressed. And because it's important to take all this information in, Master T then stuffed the instruction card into his mouth. Priceless.

At the other end in France, after carrying baby, the small suitcase, the pumps and the handbag down the stairs as the lift was broken, the porters were busy. Passengers with hands full of luggage left and soon only few people remained in the hall. I spotted a couple: he was pushing the trolley, she had her hands free. Just what I needed! Please would they would be so kind as to help me with the trolley? You should have seen her face – she looked at me as if I'd asked her to pay off my credit card. "But we are on honeymoon!" she protested. "Congratulations, that's wonderful, could you please still take my trolley out the door where I will receive help from my family? Thank you so much." Most of the passengers had cleared by now so I had no people to waste. "I will help you too," I heard, as a woman came forward, announcing to her family she'd meet them on the other side. Entourage sorted.

Anders (Thomas' father) and I then rolled the gear to the car. Next adventure: to fit it all into the Volvo Cabrio. Fitting the three suitcases and the buggy into the boot certainly deserved a high five. But it still left us with two big boxes of TPN and though one could be on the front seat, we couldn't get the other one in the back. Thomas didn't only inherit his good looks from his forebears, there is some serious logistical genius going round: Anders took all the suitcases back out, let the roof open, had me sit in the car, loaded the blue box on top of me, closed the roof and fitted the rest back in. Job done. Admittedly not exactly how I imagined riding in a Cabriolet, but we arrived safely and my newly flattened thighs suit me well.

If you are expecting any more drama or complication updates, you'll be disappointed because what followed was pure bliss. Sunshine, grandparents besotted with the Tuff, and time to snooze for me. My eyes would get tired within 30 minutes of waking up, but I suspect there was a lot of pent-up fatigue that needed to surface. I enjoyed a gorgeous view over the mountains, which turn blue in the mist of dawn and dusk. After a week I was rested enough to start thinking in clear sentences and even engage in my yoga practice. Mountain pose in front of the mountains – what harmony!

My holiday idyll was complete with laughter, pool time, and effortless team work on the TPN set-up and take-off. Great company. We had champagne and oysters and sunshine. We bought chic outfits from the French baby boutiques in Cannes, so Tuffel will be getting rather fashionable this autumn. Truly happy days. Who would have thought after all this, we'd be laughing together in such style? I am one lucky lady..

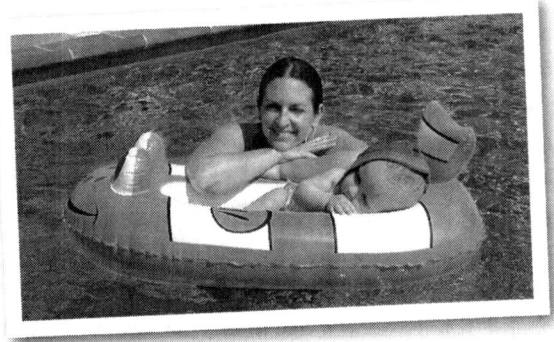

CHAPTER 16

Trust your gut

(9 MONTHS)

We were meant to get activated on the transplant list in September. It's now October.

Our next big chapter was going to be 'the wait'. Waiting for the call to let us know we had an organ. Once active on the list, we wouldn't be allowed to be more than an hour's distance from the hospital. We were going to live a waiting game, maybe for years, because the donor needs to be a baby who is Tuffel's age. But instead, our lovely transplant coordinator has stepped down.

What?

You might remember my quest to have Tuffy's bowel status rechecked, with the surgeon arguing, "But you are asking for a miracle!" My reply at the time, which surprised even me in its firmness, was: "Yes, I am". The result, to my disappointment, was that nothing had changed.

When we got to King's Hospital, our consultant gastroenterologist suggested a recheck again – both the top bit and bottom end of what Tuffel had. So we fed slightly radioactive liquid into his micro-colon. It doesn't hurt him, there are no nerves. It just turns Tuffel into a handy little nightlight, which is very useful if you are afraid of the dark.

The radiographer then screened the path of the liquid. "So this is his micro-colon then," I commented, attempting a conversation. What I saw was quite a lot of looping rather than a sorry little line to the rectum that I expected. "Micro?" she said, taking the bait, "I wouldn't call that micro-colon. It looks like a normal-sized colon to me and a bit of small bowel".

A bit of WHAT?

Apparently the structure is a bit different there at the top, and there is some 'terminal ileum'. Thank God I'm versed in the language now – if you didn't know better, wouldn't you rather *not* have terminal ileum? It sounds fatal! But it's actually very good news: it's the end of the small bowel. That part that we all thought Tuffel had zero of.

A few hours later, a very excited Dr. Hind burst into our room to talk about a possible promotion from 'no-gut' to 'short gut' and an operation to reconnect the two ends. This would mean Tuffel could lose the drainage bag and the stoma bag and would be really Wi-Fi. Well, in the daytime. We would still recharge him (with his TPN) at night. Like an iPhone. But with a bigger scream.

Reconnecting would give his gut the best chance to grow further, and who knows how much it could do? Who knows, maybe we could reduce the artificial nutrition over time… maybe we could one day come off it and he'd be 'normal'? He'd always have a shorter gut – okay, okay, that's loose stools by default, but there is now talk of healing! Talk of an option to go WITHOUT a transplant? There is now official talk of what we have been dreaming of. Of what was deemed completely impossible.

How could this happen? Did they oversee it in the beginning, or did it just grow? Was it through all the prayers, wishes, the distant healing? Was it the spirulina shakes I had taken (chlorophyll transports oxygen through the blood and promotes cell growth) to produce superfood breastmilk – had the green moustache paid off? Or was it the ingenious re-feeding? Did it really matter?

I had been re-feeding the output from the drainage bag into his fistula (the red button now covered by his stoma bag) religiously, every four hours. It was messy and time consuming. It meant emptying milky green liquid from a bag into a bowl, taking some up with a syringe into another bowl, adding some fibre powder and reinserting that mixture into his colon. I had access to his colon through the 'red button'. The beginning of Tuffel's colon had been surgically brought to the skin surface, which looks like a red button. Does that sound disgusting? I suppose if it weren't my son I would have been uncomfortable with the sight of it, but now I've seen that and so much worse. This re-feeding process has not been done much before. I have trained numerous nurses to do so, too. Jonathan (Dr. Hind) had suggested we do this to challenge the micro-colon to work and therefore to grow. You know what it's like: use it or lose it. And now we were reaping some clear, miraculous benefits from our work!

This story was slowly turning into a Hollywood movie and I liked it. Happy ending all the way, and a good portion of romance, please. I'll even have the moderate sex scenes. Actually, skip the moderate.

So for now we are not going on the transplant list. Instead we are waiting for a date to stitch Tuffy back together. This will happen in the next month or so. It's not a small operation, admittedly, but it will achieve two things: (1) connect his bowel so it is one piece and (2) tell us exactly what and how much he's got now.

A month after we heard the good news we met with the professor surgeon, who thought it wise to deflate our balloon of optimism (or rather burst it) by telling us he couldn't make out any small bowel on the ultrasound images and, even if there was now some small bowel, because it's still so little and nobody has ever had that little bowel before, he didn't see any chance for Tuffel to come off the artificial nutrition without a transplant. My energy barometer crashed. This was sobering verging on depressing! So was this all a fluke? Would our happy hopes get destroyed? What's the point in all this up and down and…?

And then we realised: nothing has changed! This is the power of thought creating our 'reality'. One 'result' telling us the miracle is happening and we are flying. Hooray! I knew it: deep inside I wished it. I've always believed in the power of love, healing and the Tuffelmeister. He's being held so dear by so many people around the world, something good was bound to happen – yippee!

Then it takes only one person to say it's not real and it all goes up in a puff of smoke. Oh no, what a disappointment.

But nothing has changed! Tuffel is still Tuffel and he's perfect as he is. With or without a bowel. The love I have for that little boy is real. The story around it can change like the weather – and it's not real, it's just a story.

So here is our lesson: keeping him in the highest vision makes us feel good and emanates joy to him. Accepting him – whatever the length of his bowel – means loving him for what he is. He doesn't have to grow a bowel in order to please me. I just want him to have a wonderful life. I would love it if it is a long and wonderful life.

I don't know how much we really choose our conditions, our physical challenges. On some days I like the idea that the soul chooses a body to express itself best in, on others I just think here we are and what happens to our body isn't all fair. Life is life and nature isn't always kind. Tuffel didn't do anything to deserve his condition.

I do believe that our inner world is reflected in our outer world, but I don't think a baby consciously chooses its external conditions. I like to believe Tuffel got himself a good deal landing himself a loving family and that we were chosen to give him all the love he needs. But I'm aware that other babies who also need a lot of love don't necessarily get it. It's not that I'm not 'chosen' to love them! I resonate with the idea of an intelligence behind life. We can only figure it out so far… the heart beats and therefore we live. But what makes it beat in the first place? Why do we suddenly breathe?

I believe in love; I believe in miracles. I don't believe in a person called God, I believe in the energy of creation flowing through us. I call that energy God or Love. I believe I could go and give a sermon now, but I'm tired and should sleep. I tend to lecture in my head a lot between 3am and 4am – if you'd like to tune into my thoughts just after nappy changing, I come up with pretty deep stuff, man.

So where were we? At the gospel of Tuff: Trust your gut. And allow the miracles to unfold from there.

CHAPTER 17
Everybody needs a Bridget
(8 MONTHS)

As part of our complex discharge planning, we were introduced to Carrie, the continuing care nurse for Lambeth. I call her Carrie Carepackage because she arranges our continuing health care home package. It is really incredible thinking about it: The locally governed NHS (national health service) called CCG, which was called PCT before, confuses the heck out of any community member. But apart from that, it pays for our continuing care package. In short, for nurses to come to our home and help as it's not really possible to leave us with the whole weight of Tuffel's 24-hour care requirements. There is a lot of paperwork being done and I'm glad it's not on my shoulders. Carrie is also sorting out our home TPN. What a blessing to have such an efficient force of nature in the team. Carrie works in a temporary position. She should be employed if you ask me. They couldn't find a better person and the PCCTV NHS local trust would save money they could spend on brainstorming more departments with clever abbreviations shortening names nobody understands. If they saved their money at the right places, would they need to be as tight on the care packages? Thank God. In America we'd need a pretty good insurance to cover us. As I now know, not everyone has that and people run into serious financial distress trying to keep their children alive. As a UK taxpayer, I don't have to worry about this. Incredible. To give you an idea, a daily feed of TPN costs around £100.

I never thought I'd receive so much help or that I'd be in need of receiving so much help.

She doesn't like me calling her Carrie Carepackage, but I'm sure she understands it's a great way to remember her name. I have so many people in my life now doing so many things for our little boy, I'm glad if I know my own name and role by the end of each day.

I was briefed not to be too positive so she would see that we need help and we wouldn't want to be cut short because of my resilience and optimism. It turned out I didn't need to put on an act because she got it anyway. She understood that strong people can be left behind in the support system because they are 'coping well'. Which doesn't mean they don't deserve a helping hand in tough situations.

It had been evaluated that we'd get eight hours of nursing help every week. Thomas and I would have a say in which provider would get the contract to deliver those eight hours of care. I spoke to three nursing providers. The first one was the biggest one and the rep reminded me of an insurance salesman. It was a bit awkwardly formal. When I asked if I would meet the nurses first, I was told that wasn't possible. But if I wasn't happy with what I got, they could possibly change her. Would you leave your child in the hands of a stranger? Turns out that TPN-trained nurses are a bit of a rarity anyway, so we wouldn't be left with too many choices. A promising start.

The second nursing company hadn't really read the brief and started selling us carers. They didn't even ask what Tuffel needed, so that was an easy rejection to make. And the third provider was a small and personable company that sounded as if they were going to do anything to help us out. We'd meet the nurses and would choose which one we liked, they were flexible in hours and I had access to the director 24/7. Thomas and I love small, personable businesses so the decision was made.

Two weeks later and we still hadn't started our package. I grew more and more tired. Three weeks passed. I am a powerhouse but by then my batteries were running low. After a month I think we had the first nurse scheduled to start, but because she worked elsewhere during the day, it had to be an evening shift. Thomas had bought us tickets to an event on happiness. We were ready to go, suited and booted. Time to go. No nurse in sight. Phone calls were made, stress levels rising…The nurse was 20 minutes late. We weren't very happy. Spot the irony. We'd missed our opportunity to go out. After getting rid of our annoyance, we decided to still take some time out. So an overtired couple left the house without any plans and four hours on their hands. Painting the town red.

I remember us buying a cheap vodka cranberry at our local store in order to get drunk on Clapham Common. We had to do something. What we wanted was sleep. But it was too cold on the Common for that. Feeling like teenagers, pretending we liked the drink when really, cranberry juice alone would have been much nicer, we danced around on the grass to keep warm, feeling a bit sheepish. Then we discovered we could play darts in a local pub; we kept ourselves busy until we were 'allowed' back home. Nights out are a great idea in principle. But when you haven't slept through in 10 months, knowing you've got the night shift ahead, it's just not the same.

Then we had a weekend nurse booked. She didn't turn up. We had no notice. Nothing. Never mind, I didn't have any plans anyway – besides sleeping – and the director was so apologetic, it left me feeling sorry for her and the nurse. Who knows what had happened to her! After a while we had two night nurses: one was lovely, cleaning Tuffel's cupboard in her downtime, the other one was content to watch our telly for four hours! When I got home, I'd hang up the washing, fold the dry clothes and do the dishes. Exhausted. Is it too much to ask a person in your house with four free hours on their hands, who gets paid a fair wage, to help out? Because as it turns out there are four hours in the day during which Tuffel is the easiest boy in the world: between 7pm and 11pm.

Anyway, daytime nurses would start soon. Promises, promises. I met one nurse available for the job. But after trying to educate me that watching TV was indeed educational, when I had made it clear that I didn't want Tuffel to watch telly – and not spending a single minute engaging with Tuffel during her entire interview, she was already in my bad books. After an hour, she asked me what my name was. I put my foot down and one of the directors herself was going to come and take over for the time being. But she got ill. So another three weeks passed until Thomas had had enough and did the manly thing of contacting Carrie and firing the agency.

A new player had arrived and was eager to take the opportunity of his first paediatric contract. Amit, representing Bespoke Agency, is a nice guy and I was keen to see if he could deliver. Instead of wading through his books to find a match, he'd advertise and hire people just for us. That sounded much more sensible. Turned out rather challenging though. But Carrie, being the proactive soul that she is, made a few phone calls around her respectable colleagues and before long we had a team of nurses that came highly recommended. Everyone was happy.

I now know that many families with care packages struggle to find suitable carers and nurses because unfortunately carers don't get paid well and there aren't many paediatric nurses working freelance on zero-hour contracts. We now have a wonderful team with Angela, Carol and Bridget. My favourite nurse is Bridget, who really is way too senior for the job, but that's not the point. The point of being an agency nurse is to keep your clinical skills up and do some actual nursing rather than whatever high rank administrative role she might have worked herself up to.

Agency work can be well paid, especially with a good little company like Bespoke. It's important that staff get paid well; it shows in their reliability and motivation. Bridget has decades of experience and also knows everyone in the sector. She has four kids: two biologically her own, two adopted. She came into our little messy flat and just started sorting things out. She'll do some ironing when Tuffel is sleeping, hang up washing and take him to all sorts of fun activities. She knows more playgroups in Clapham than I do and finds new places to go and explore. She took him to Godsted farm, Hyde park, the museum and soft play. With her, I have no doubt Tuffel has a great time and, most importantly, he is safe. We can't just let him be with anybody. If something was to happen, you need to know exactly what to do. When we have a question, she most likely has an answer or knows who to ask. Everyone is revived when Bridget is around. Tuffel loves her. The big smile on his face when she comes shows it clearly and he happily gives her kisses and cuddles.

Obviously Bridget doesn't have much time. It has been worth the long wait to have Bridget in our lives. As time progressed and the nights got harder, we were allocated more hours: 12. I am eternally grateful for those 12 hours. They make a huge difference. When we have a house, it would be good to get night care. Getting up two to 12 times each night isn't easy and some rest would be appreciated. But my allocated 12 hours covers one night… so it's more helpful to use them in the daytime, as it can cover two days. It allows me to do a yoga class and some work. I thought I'd be resting and recovering in these breaks but it turns out that that's not good enough for me. I get quite frustrated in the rut of childcare and recovery, nursing, being a mummy, resting, and housework. I feel a strong need to contribute to other people's lives outside my family. I want to be part of society, express my creativity, develop professionally, and generate money. I detest the idea of doing the washing in 'my' time. Or shopping. These tasks can be done with Tuffel. My break is for things that I just need concentration for: writing articles, coaching, giving workshops and talks. Admin and emails. Life is a lot better with Bridget around.

Home life is wonderful, all in all. Thomas has said he finally feels like a proper family. He feels paternal now. This is the stuff not spoken about so much, but bonding with your child is not a given. It has to happen somewhere and it was challenging to become a 'parent' emotionally when we had to take a bus to visit this child of ours. We both found it weird and I spent as little time as possible thinking about it. I just did what I needed to do. Over time this new day-to-day became my normal and I accepted the wired bundle as my kid – in a way I talked myself into it – it wasn't a 100% instinctive bond initially. I can say that after having him home for a while we feel a strong bond and we feel like very proud parents indeed.

I remember when I got ill once and had to stay away from the ward for three days I felt so guilty because I didn't miss him. Am I a bad mother? I had cooked a lovely oven dish, testing it after 25 minutes, only deciding it needed a little longer. I had completely forgotten that tasting an egg-based meal early would not be a good idea. The next day I didn't feel so good. Well, you can imagine this is an understatement and also what came next. I was banned from going anywhere near the hospital as the rules state that anyone with vomiting and diarrhoea has to stay clear to prevent the spread of viruses such as Norovirus. Instead I had myself the lousiest 48 hours since being giving birth!

I was shivering and decided to take a bath. Then I felt faint so I got out. The runs set in. So with my trademark breast pump in hand (as warm water stimulates lactation) I was in a serious pump or spray-all-over-the-place dilemma, but as a woman I thought I could multitask. What was I thinking? Naked, faint, shivering and wet woman with breast pump on the loo. Nice image. Suddenly I was overcome with the urge to hurl at the same time. Had I not been so ill, this was the point I would have laughed. It was too ridiculously disgusting. Lucky I wasn't on my first date.

When Thomas asked me how I felt, not having seen my little miracle man in two days, all I could say was "empty" – pun and no pun, with no rush to get back to St Thomas' hospital. I didn't miss him. I didn't want to see him. I felt guilty about it. A mother should always want to be with her baby, surely. I should be wanting to get well and get back to the cot! I just wanted to sleep and not go anywhere. Ever.

This was my lesson to be kind and compassionate to myself and not to expect what I think society tells me to do. Life is often different from what one expects.

All this seems so far away now. Since having our boy home, we are a real family. We laugh, cuddle and live. We don't test egg-based meals too early. We feel good. We have help that works. We have each other and we have Bridget. These are happy days.

CHAPTER 18

Opening up

(10 MONTHS)

We are going back to hospital on Tuesday (14th November) to have Tuffel's bowel connected by surgery. Yes, it is exciting. It's positive.

Interestingly enough that's not how we've felt of late…

We've really had enough of being hospitalised. And here we are entering uncertainty yet again. Only when they cut him open all across his tummy will we know what we've really got. Only then will they know if they can actually connect, or if they would leave him with a stoma (a surgically created exit for his waste). Which would be an even messier affair than what I'm currently dealing with (I have a drainage bag through his belly that empties what lands in the stomach and I change stoma bags around his red button thingy – the entry point to his colon). I'm a girl, I like a nice bag, but stoma bags just don't cut it for me. Should I ask Prada to make some?

We really wish for him to get rid of the bags and fistula on his body. In the best case scenario, he'll be left with only the central line for his TPN feed. He could eat any kind of food. It would be amazing! So far we could feed him puree but we have to be careful not to block his tubes. The doctors are always worried about anything getting stuck in his dead-end pouch of a duodenum. We can't afford things to get infected in there.

I'm dreading the 'straight talk' from the doctors, who have to tell us every gory risk involved. I feel I've held the space for miracles well. And now I am so tired. Tired of trying not to go to that painful place inside myself, tired of it still sneaking into my awareness through my dreams at night.

I'd like to not 'go there'. 'There' being the fear of what could go wrong. 'There' being the sorrow of seeing him with wounds and sedated for days or weeks. Nobody can tell us how long it will be until he comes home again. 'There' being the terrifying feeling that comes with signing his life away, accepting all risks and their consequences before each operation. It's one of the hardest things to do. Well it's not hard to do, it's just a signature as long as nothing goes wrong. If it did, the signature turns into a responsibility. And it's hard to take responsibility for something we do not control that is so important.

I've gotten to know this little boy so well. I love him so much. I am attached to him.

I don't want to go there.

I want to be in a positive mood. I want to stay in the now, in the moment, in the 'here we are and we have him and we love being together'. Though I must confess that being in the now sometimes means 'I am so tired because you kept me up half the night blowing raspberries and gurgling and crying'. Living in the now is much better when the 'now' is pleasant.

So what do you do when life just doesn't work that way?

The other night, Thomas and I were supposed to see *Skyfall* at the cinema, but I didn't get tickets. After a stupid argument about how I should have found somewhere other than the local cinema, with me explaining that I was running an hour late all day, we realised that arguing takes a lot of time. Time would be wasted if invested in arguing. We could be watching *The X Factor*! Think what you may about this program, it is a great distraction from our daily routines.

As this penny dropped, we gave up on our argument. Sadly, *The X Factor* doesn't screen on Fridays, so instead we immersed ourselves in a beautifully connective chat, sharing our vulnerability about the upcoming operation. I hadn't opened up like that in a while. Not even when my mum was over to help. I felt too tired, too busy, too stressed. I just didn't feel I had the time for tears. I don't want to spend my time on crying. It makes me tired and I need every ounce of energy I can muster.

In other words I was too caught up in my 'own little world'. I didn't realise how I was cutting myself off from my inner peace, limiting my daily experience to such a degree. Instead I have suffered from blocked sinuses and felt that I didn't have much to talk about. I felt disconnected somewhere, but I couldn't tell where. It felt rather dissatisfying.

And I've had nightmare after nightmare. In one dream I experienced Tuffel dying from a freak disease that my bowel specialists just didn't know about and nonchalantly said, "Hmm, we don't know," as his flesh was slowly detaching from his bones.

I suppose my dreams of late have been the perfect build-up to Halloween. I was hoping for treats, but instead my mind was playing tricks on me and I fell for it. Over and over and over again, taking my thoughts seriously, wading through the mud of such mental morass.

In another dream, blood soaked through the sheets as his line had been pulled out. A horror emergency scenario unfolds. In that dream I struggled to remember what I needed to do and my head was so blurry, my movements slow and frazzled as blood ran out of his little body, leaving him paler by the second. Was I to call the ambulance first or disinfect? Clamp the line! Oh yes, that's right: I have to clamp at the closest point to him so he can't bleed out – but where is the clamp?

As much as I have been disappointed about broken dreams before, now I am grateful when they don't follow through to the end. And I appreciate that not all dreams come true. What a relief.

And last night, in a state of sleeplessness – courtesy of my blocked nasal passages – I had an epiphany. After watching a video of Mara Gleason and Aaron Turner of the One Thought Institute, which specialises in unlocking human potential, I realised: a nightmare is just thinking. I can ask at any time for another thought. Thoughts really aren't real. Deal me another card (another thought). Thanks. I was trying to figure out how to express my fears more in the daytime to avoid the nightmares; but I don't have to do anything to change my thoughts in the day. There is no need for that when I see that these thoughts are just part of my personal thinking. Life is bigger than my personal thinking and that reconnects me to my wellbeing.

Speaking means expressing my thoughts. But thought expressions don't equate reality creation as much as some 'law of attraction' gurus want us to believe. If it were true, most of us would have died in an airplane crash. Whatever is, is, and will be – regardless of how much I worry or don't worry about it. I don't have to control my thoughts to stay positive. Real positivity is much deeper than surface level reframing of thoughts. I can't necessarily avoid the nightmares by saying lots of vulnerable things in the day. I can express lots of fears and it won't guarantee me happy dreams. But if I know that dreams and thoughts aren't as real as they may feel, I can relax about the process. I'm ok even when I have bad dreams sometimes.

Meanwhile, on another level, life with Tuffel is really good. He's such a lovely, cuddly boy. Maybe he could drop the habit of waking up hourly from 2am. Thomas and I are so tired. When we are tired, clarity likes to take a nap first and negative thoughts tend to stick just that little bit more, masquerading as truths. They are still only thoughts! Obviously I wouldn't complain about happy thoughts sticking around, but as you will probably have experienced for yourself, it's often the darker ones that stick to our consciousness like superglue to your skin after an art attack session.

He's asleep. But is he alive? When I drive I quickly feel his fontanelle pulse. In the buggy, I await a twitch or I poke him. The other day he freaked me out with a stare into the distance whilst not moving for what seemed forever. He didn't react to me calling him. "Tuffel!!!" That snapped him out of it – oops sorry, I didn't mean to scare you.

I didn't want to talk about my fears for a while because I don't like it when people 'understand'. There is nothing worse than other people 'understanding' the worry and confirming it. I don't need that. Or even worse, the friendly attempts at psychological counsel. The other thing I don't like is a play-down: 'Oh, you'll be all right; I'm sure it will be fine'. It seems to be socially convenient, adapting the positive stance – after all, life must go on and we don't want to leave a conversation on a low.

All that's really needed is the space to be myself in. Since having allowed the pain out by confiding in Thomas, I've been feeling more real, more alive, more me again. I even wrote an open-hearted email to my mum. Deep honesty is the key to my livelihood. It's the bravest, deepest, coolest and most rewarding gift I can give myself.

I have no idea how the next weeks/months will be. Will I sleep in hospital in a room full of screaming babies? Will being woken up by a chatting Tuffel seem more peaceful than to be woken up by screams and alarms? Will I be able to go home and come back in the morning without him missing us too much? How long will it be? Will he be healing fast? Will he be on monitors and cables again? Oh gee, I don't miss seeing him like that... We've come so far.

I know that Thomas and I will reconnect to the foundation of our relationship and hold hands in this. I'm tempted to say 'no matter what, we'll deal with it,' but it's not how I see it. I care deeply about the outcome of the next few weeks. This isn't about 'dealing'. I am having an intense experience and that's the truth. May it be a rich experience. What I am asking for is inner peace and guidance – and the growth which is the underlying gift of all challenges.

CHAPTER 19
How to make a miracle

(10 MONTHS)

Tuffel has had his operation, and we're in the Rays of Sunshine ward, where the nurses are lovely, the doctors handsome and the cases hardcore. Third liver transplant; kids from all over the world; an unknown disease that has left a toddler without any immune system, but with a bowel that forms stomas by itself (?!). Our six-month old smiley cot neighbour could have been saved by a single blood test. But the health professionals had not been concerned about the bit of yellow in the eyes. Now she needs a new liver to survive. One baby in our room died two days ago.

Rays of Sunshine... where the sun don't shine and if it does we can't see it because the view sucks.

But the sun is in all our hearts. This is an exemplary children's hospital with the most caring staff. We've been here for over a week nonstop. I've left the building twice: for yoga and ballroom dancing. I hear one goes mad after a while living in hospital, but the good news is it feels good! I put cold water on my teabag and wondered why it wasn't getting brown. I didn't comprehend why nurse Becca was here at 8am when she'd been in yesterday! I figured it out eventually: she'd gone home overnight! Ahh, yes. Time for a mad chicken dance...

My nurse, apparently, was still in hangover. I thought that was rather unprofessional until I computed they meant the *hand*over. And I told one nurse I really wanted to get rid of this staff! I meant stuff.

The operation itself went well. But it came with bad news. We had so hoped for bowel to have grown. It had all looked so promising. The idea was to lengthen whatever was there and work it from there. We were prepared for the op to last up to six hours. After four hours we got the call: alas, there was no bowel to lengthen. It's official. Tuffel has no small intestine. None.

Where is our miracle?

He's now got his duodenum stitched to his colon, so whatever goes into his mouth will come out of his bottom. The next question will be how fast and how furiously. Bottom management is our new mission. I'll print it on my business cards. Evelyne Brink: Author, Coach and Bottom Management Specialist.

First things first. Seven days of no food, no drink. He watches me eat, but he makes no fuss. The day after the operation he was sitting up in his cot, playing. Day two, we're smiling again. After four days we took the epidural out. Followed by the catheter in his willy; the nose tube followed the next day. After six days he let go of all painkillers. Children are amazing! We live in the nursery with a changing cast of ill babies. I am thriving in my position of experienced hospital mum, giving support, perspective and nursery rhyme concerts to the newcomers.

One evening after a particularly mad day, I tucked little Meister into his hospital blanket and sang my repertoire of international nursery rhymes. When he had dropped off,

I peeked through the curtains to find all the babies and parents present in the room fast asleep! En-chanted.

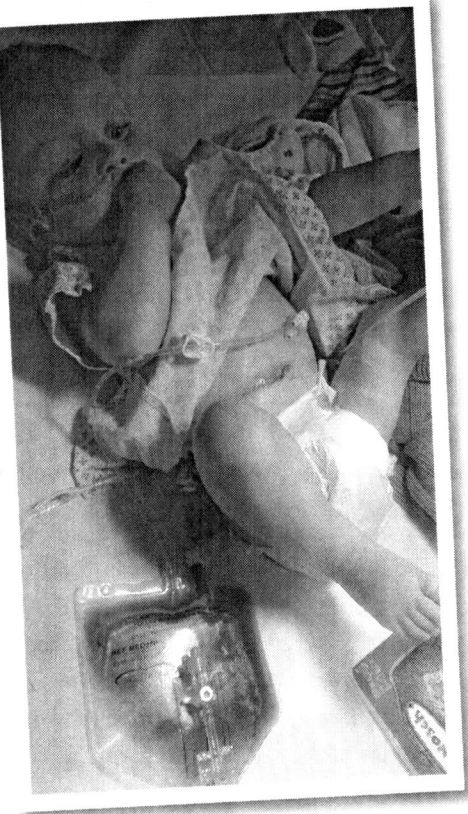

(In case you're wondering about the bag in this post-op picture, it's just for the initial stage of recovery... when a bowel gets operated on, it does what French postmen are known for: goes on strike for a few days. So we are draining the stomach. This is the bag that is going to disappear! Along with the 'red button' stoma, which is now gone.)

One baby had no mum at her side after being rolled in, post-op. What kind of mother leaves her beautiful nine-week old alone? We were raging. I bought the little one a balloon. She had nothing! I sang for her behind the curtain. I'm not allowed to touch. I could feel people's anger at the mum. I could feel my different emotions: how could she? It left me angry and sad, but choosing to consider that this mum must have a reason felt more true, and made me feel curious and peaceful. I asked the nurse: turns out the mum was stuck in Ireland without a visa. Poor mother! When I told the other mums, their faces softened instantly. Interesting how thought creates feeling and how a new feeling takes over as soon as perspective changes. Two days later, baby's mum finally arrived. Gracious and so grateful that we had taken care of her child. We had a good time and I hope they had a lovely journey back home.

Tuffel loves his stethoscope. I'm not a fan of those all flashing, singing electronic plastic constructions sold as 'toys' anyway. I love T discovering and developing his lovely, sensitive nature. Luckily, the play therapist here likes me and she went on a search for some wooden toys and books. But then again, with a blood pressure machine, a red-light pulse probe and a stethoscope, who needs toys? Plus, we have two oranges and a cardboard bowl. He's loving it.

I might sound positive, but underneath we were saddened by the news of Tuffel's missing bowel. With all the prayers and blessings and healing sessions and visualising... well... as much as we'd like to think we can make miracles happen, some things have their own way. We don't manipulate the world. Interesting lesson.

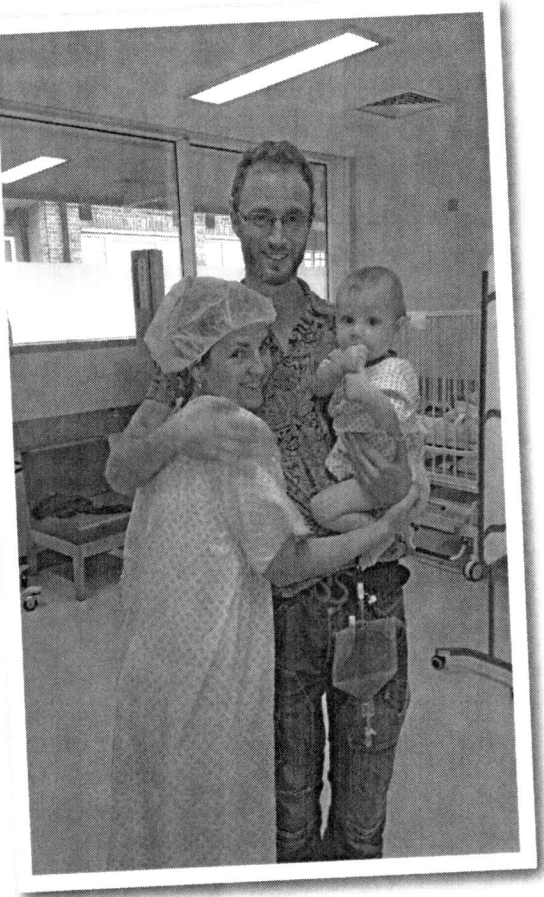

Then Thomas had a lightbulb moment. Ping!

If we aren't getting a miracle from upstairs, let's create one ourselves. Thomas has launched himself into a researching frenzy, finding that medical advances have opened up brilliant possibilities. Stem cells could be the solution, or perhaps a new way to avoid the need for immunosuppressant drugs. The scary thing about transplants are the drugs one has to live on afterwards – which are so poisonous you have to wear a mask preparing them. If things can progress quickly enough so that Tuffel can benefit from stem cell research – that would be amazing.

So Thomas is in the process of setting up our own charity to raise money for research. Many children (and adults) need transplants and new organs and they all will benefit from better ways to manage replacement parts. We have amazing friends who are helping us: Sam Harvey is donating his film-making skills to make an explanatory video, Thomas' friend Max is brainstorming fundraising ideas. Sarah-Louise Young will look into bucket collections. We may stage a charity concert.

So yes... making our own miracle. Watch this space.

CHAPTER 20

Christmas gagagadada style

(11 MONTHS)

Thomas and I took a little walk in the Bedfordshire countryside. We've taken this walk many times – whenever we visit Thomas' Auntie Inge in her cosy Swedish-style cottage. But usually the fields aren't this flooded and usually my eyes aren't this wet either. A happy/ relieved/ what-the-f***k cry. It's been a year since our last visit. And what a year it has been.

After all we've been through and how much we've grown this year, we are here: a family reunited with our little super baby, celebrating 'Chrissemas' – as Thomas pronounces it. Danish cookies, flags on the tree, roasted duck with red cabbage, apples, oranges and prunes. Presents on Christmas Eve. Dancing around the tree, singing carols too loudly: come ooon, it's Chrissemas.

It was always going to be special to see this time of year through our child's eyes. The shine, the curiosity, this infectious joy has given me so many heart-warming moments already and it was enhanced by Tuffel's wondrous gazing at the tree, the lights, and the big family gathering. "Gagaga! Dadada," Tuffel delights in the sweetest voice.

All this year I held back from expectations and fantasies about the future. But admittedly, when we went back to hospital last month, our goal was to get him out before the festivities. It wasn't a 'SMART' (specific, measurable, realistic, time-bound) goal we find in the classic coaching toolkit as it really wasn't in our hands. We were prepared to stay there for up to three months. But Tuffel is great, we proved ourselves reliable enough to continue his cares at home, and so we were discharged after the minimum time of two weeks. Apart from that, guess what: I don't really do SMART goals these days. They just can't hold up with reality and its infinite possibilities.

In stark contrast to the "We're so sorry, we don't think he'll make it" we were told over the cot of a highly wired-up neonate in Intensive Care at the beginning of this year, we achieved a happy family Christmas at home, wireless during the day with the cutest and happiest boy the hospital has known. Wow. Just stick a bow on him – I couldn't ask for a better present.

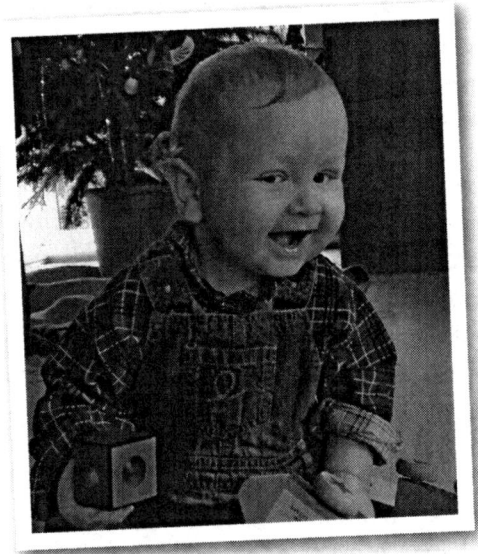

I have noticed that our conversations may not have been particularly deep or memorable of late. I do sometimes yearn for passionate discussions, but the main content of my verbal expressions these days revolves around: "Isn't he cute… He's too cute… OMG he's just too cute." Sometimes I do wonder whether the rest of my vocabulary will eventually return. Suffice to say, as restricted as my output may be, at least it feels good. The other bonus? Thomas and I agree. And there isn't that much more to say than: "Tuffel – sooo cuute!"

Although we have learned a new expression over Christmas: "Woopa – Gangnam style! " Yes, thanks to Tuffel's cousins, Scarlett and Daisy, (nine and seven years old) we have finally caught up on pop culture and viral videos. Thomas' legendary performance of the Gangnam dance became a definite highlight of our festivities.

The nights have been tough. Since they connected the upper part of his bowel (the duodenum) to the lowest part (the colon), Tuffmeister's stool output has increased to a whopping seven to nine stools daily, with a record of 14. Most of these happen at night and due to their unprocessed nature, they act like a chemical peel. Against the already delicate skin of a baby's bottom. We are waging a constant battle against red rectums and burnt balls. That means getting up in the night at the smallest sound to check and change him, Formula 1 pit stop-style.

I've been quite tired (note my British understatement). Thomas had taken over some night shifts with Tuffel on top of his own work, he was getting rather exhausted. Christmas with the family has been as much a special celebration as a sanctuary – food magically appearing and nap times becoming available. I'm even indulging in reading a book of the light entertainment, chick-lit genre. One nobody will ever ask me about and I won't need to remember the content of, but due to its easy-reading nature, I do remember it all and then tell everyone who doesn't want to know about it.

Given that my head has been rather fuzzy lately, I'm glad I am functioning and able to just enjoy. I've even been blessed with a sprinkle of restlessness and the odd 'What am I going to do with my life?' thought. It's not as if I don't know what I want to do, but at this state of deep mum-fatigue, I don't remember that I know and I start questioning everything until my brain shuts down. Thankfully it does shut down. That's the plus side of fatigue – it stops silly thinking rather quickly via abrupt crashing. When you can't hold a sentence together, you also don't hold onto grudges, confusions about life and the helpless feelings associated with world politics.

"I didn't know you're buying a flat!" said a surprised friend last week. Probably because I forgot to mention that minor detail. We had an offer accepted while in hospital, and sitting at the cot I had been instructing lawyers and surveyors and dealing with the country's national plague – estate agents. I have never witnessed such unnecessary nuisances since my days of dealing with German bureaucracy! I am even going to make a stand for German bureaucracy at this point, as it all seems meaningful in comparison. I thought what Tuffel had was a pain in the bum, until I had to work with estate agents.

The stirring up of emotional froth thanks to all the hot air and stupidity I'd been dealing with spun my mind into the numbest state of bored panic ever. We must have had the unhappiest seller in the world, who from day one "wasn't happy" about our choice of lawyers (none of her business), leaving the agent to threaten that the deal was "dead in the water" and since then kept being "unhappy" that things were moving slowly, all the while neglecting the fact that the ball was mainly in their court. I was on the verge of sending anti-depressants with a Christmas card. No, I wasn't really. Here is our home-buying story abridged: we offered, we moved forward, we didn't get answers to our questions, we pulled out. A simple script plumped up with heavy lawyers, stressful talk, threats and endless blahblahblah.

It's easy to get sucked into upset and stress. I nearly missed out on my arts and crafts session at the hospice (every two months, Tuffel and I enjoy a few days' respite at Shooting Star Children's Hospice), talking through my property dilemma with a dad, who in turn offloaded his.

When Carrie Carepackage introduced the idea of using a hospice, my face nearly slid off my head. A hospice? No way! Isn't that where people go to die? "Think of it like a posh hotel where you get to stay for free whilst they give Tuffel a really good time," she said. "It's not just end of life care although, let's be honest, that's what they do, too. They also offer respite. They have a pool, a sensory room, lots of toys and space and one-on-one care." That did sound appealing. So now we benefit from a few nights of respite here and there and Tuffel has become their poster boy, featuring in magazines and fundraising campaigns. I never thought I'd be the one benefiting from a charity. To me charity is something you give to. Not get from. Oh, I am so grateful it exists.

And here I was wasting my precious respite time on 'what goes wrong with houses' conversations. Of course, his was much heavier, including builders who went bust whilst renovating his home for his daughter's disability and being trapped by the fact that every potential home purchase would need huge adjustments for her, as the one he's got is too small and can't be extended. This was the precise boring, problem-based adult talk I never wanted to get into! How can we get so passionate talking about such crap?

Thank goodness for the powers of glitter which lit the path back to sanity as I crafted a tea light and card for the hospice staff. I cannot commend the team here highly enough. They are amazing.

CHAPTER 21

Happy Birthday!

Is this nuts or what: one year ago I had a book launch planned (*The ARTrepreneur: Financial Success for Artistic Souls* – available on Amazon) and cancelled to prepare for the appearance of Mr T.

One year ago, after 36 hours of intensity, Tuffel Leo came to this world. The midwife said: "This was the easy part! Now the hard work begins."

She was right. But she'd never meant it *that* way. One year ago we were given the most horrific diagnosis by our doctors.

That was then.

And now here we are. Happy, proud, grateful.

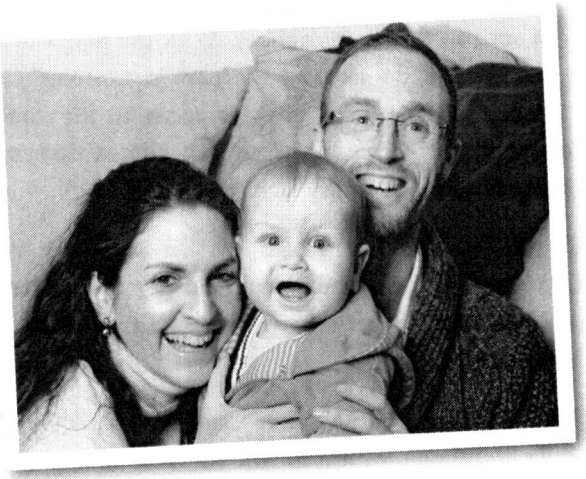

Out of hospital, healthy and miraculously well, we have a WiFi baby by day and a trendy smartbaby we plug in at night. With a bit of a leaky battery... (I'm trying to get out of talking about my baby's secretions nonstop by using metaphors instead... does it work?)

We have wonderful nurses who look after him 12 hours a week to give me a break. Bupa delivers the artificial nutrition and the many medical supplies he needs and even though there are plenty of mistakes, we always get there in the (longwinded) end.

People call it teething problems. Any parent knows that teething can be a minor deal or a major upset. There were teething problems of both kinds. Thankfully, Tuffel manages to grow his own teeth with less stress. He's got two proud new ones with three coming through at the moment. Impressive.

His bowel is all joined up from the top end to the bottom end. There may be no small intestine, but there is a whole lot of sprit in that little monkey. With the long scar line on the lower abdomen and the new gastrostomy called a 'mickey button' which gives us access to his stomach looking like a goggled eye, we can almost declare his tummy as a kind of smiley face.

We still live in our one-bedroom flat in Nappy Valley (Clapham Old Town) and it's tight but cosy. So far, I haven't found anything bigger that was better. That's reserved for the year ahead.

Tuffel makes the cutest sounds and loves cuddling. I'm loving it beyond pancakes. It's the best feeling in the world. I was prepared to experience a deeper love than ever, a magical bond, the whole cheese. And as always, understanding an idea intellectually and experiencing it in your body are two completely different things. You can see it my eyes, energy, in my inability to form complete sentences at a time. I've reinvented myself a fair few times before, but this experience is transformative at root level. Transformative in that it's brought my loving core to the forefront. And with that, the world looks and feels different.

The whole silly silent worries of 'What if he turns out to be a criminal later? What if my son was a bully? Would I still love him? Can I love him now thinking *that*?' I had entertained in pregnancy when I didn't have bigger things to worry about yet… they've completely dissolved. I'm way too busy enjoying the moment. And if I haven't mentioned it yet: he's too cute! When he grows up he'll think his name is 'Awwwwtoocuuuute'!

My little hero is into books and wooden toys. He seems to agree with the 'no noisy toys' policy under my roof, happily gravitating towards simple, beautifully crafted playthings himself. I don't mean to be dogmatic, but my passion on this topic amuses even me: I don't like the plastic 'supporting the development of your child' kind of imagination-killers. If you feel like winding me up, get me started on it.

He likes to laugh at random times. Unexpectedly, when the mood hits. A trait I myself had to learn to control over time (it doesn't seem to be appreciated amongst adults). Finally – someone who justifies my interrupting serious meetings or breaking up the day with a bit of a laughing fit. Hooray!

I've always known that having a kid is the ultimate excuse for being yourself. I run through the supermarket with him riding in the trolley and I skate with my feet pulled by the speed of the trolley – how naughty and fun. I get to dance and sing loudly wherever I want. Before, people might have thought I was strange going on desperate. I'm not denying that – but, curiously, that very behaviour is now classified as 'being a good mum'. Though the 'mum' label is still not the sexiest brand in society, I wear it like a Jimmy Choo shoe. Proud and trying not to show the pain.

No matter how expensive your stilts, they are still a strange construction to put under one's foot, trying to balance a body on a planet that spins at some 1000 miles per hour. I'm watching Tuffel practising his standing, and am reminded how much goes into it! We take it for granted now unless we're completely ramshackled (that's drunk, for non-British readers). That's when standing up reverts back to its original miraculousness. I digress...

So one year... to help us celebrate, we'll have family over from Germany and Denmark, Cambridge, Bedford and even my 94-year-old Great Aunt, Tuffel's Greatest Aunt, will come all the way from West London.

They WILL come. They will come... will they? My mum has been stuck at the airport all day and will attempt to fly in via Geneva in the early hours. Thomas' parents are travelling from France and hope to make it to Gatwick – the snow has disrupted so much, I've started eating the big chilli I'd precooked for everyone's arrival.

CHAPTER 22

The big One

(12 MONTHS)

Our apartment is really too small for everyone I've invited, but I convinced myself it was going to be okay. The loo queue would be similar to the ladies' during interval at a West End theatre production. I would sing to distract the crowd from their aching full bladders. I bought balloons and even green paper cups and – wait for it – matching napkins. Professional event planning all the way.

My mother embarked on an epic adventure from Frankfurt, lingering at the airport for a day, flying out to Geneva next morning as Heathrow airport had been closed. I think someone had farted in the wrong direction and they were too embarrassed to admit that it brought the planes to a standstill. They said it was the snow. So she was diverted to London City but that closed, too.

My suspicion: someone working at that airport had the same meal.

Anyway, they flew her to Heathrow, which had by this point reopened. Her suitcase was eventually found and, as the tube wasn't working, (maybe a Tic Tac mint had fallen on the track; those little dispensers are sometimes hard to control) she took a bus to Hammersmith and the underground from there.

You'd expect her to be exhausted and annoyed from the 48-hour trip, but she proved just why she's so incredible. When she arrived, she excitedly recalled her adventure, during which she befriended a Nigerian Lawyer from Norway and discussed the concept of identity with a young man from South Africa, who runs a language school in Heidelberg. I love my mum.

Thomas' parents had flown in from France, somehow having gotten the only flight with no delays. That's the Westenholzes summed up for you. The world might be in chaos, Tic Tacs on train lines, gassy bowels closing airports, but it doesn't seem to affect them. I love my outlaws.

Our family situated in England didn't make it.

It was too dangerous for my 94-year-old Great Aunt to walk outside. The Cambridge/Bedford branch of the family had to turn around as the snow on the unlit roads made it too dangerous to drive. They were as gutted as were we. We had a conversation via satellite instead. Amazing that it would be easier to shoot signals through space than to see each other.

We cancelled the musical chairs game and loo-queue entertainment and celebrated a magically intimate family birthday. My mum's loud laughter made for some joyously nutty nutcake baking. Tuffel loved his day. He was in great spirits and enjoyed all the attention. It was so heart-warming, all the airports reopened the next day!

So now he's a year old, I thought it's time to do something for me again.

I gave my first talk on my book, *The ARTrepreneur*, for the Surviving Actors event in Portland Square last Saturday.

What a surreal experience to stand in front of a room again speaking. The content of my book seemed so far away. I really enjoyed when the information flooded my brain again and working with people on the spot is simply joyful.

When I checked my phone, Thomas had left five desperate messages. Not now! Tuffel wasn't well, his temperature had risen and the usually bonny boy was crying nonstop. I rushed home and, to cut a long story short, we had to take him to hospital for a suspected line infection. That's what it's like for Tuffel each time he shows a temperature. They administered two strong antibiotics four times a day. Blood tests, cannulas that fell out, more needles. He also needed a blood transfusion as he hasn't produced enough red blood cells. The temperature spike could just be due to teething. But with a central line, we can't afford that kind of thinking. Bacteria in the line would be flushed into the top heart chamber and spread throughout his entire bloodstream and the organs it supplies in no time.

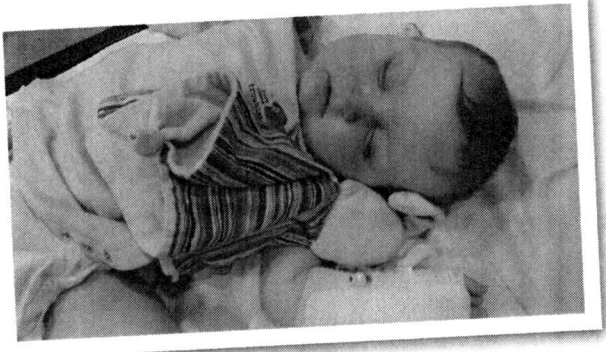

Combining motherhood of Tuffel and my own wishes to grow as an author and coach look like a real challenge from the outside. Was this episode a sign that it just wouldn't work? Would I always have to rush out of my opportunities to attend emergencies? Is it really 'me or him'? It's so easy to read into situations and make meaning out of them. It's so easy to buy into fear. When I listen more deeply, I get the feeling these two facets of my life will come together beautifully. I don't know when and I don't know how. I will keep hanging out in that familiar place that is the unknown.

Taking each day at a time for the gift that it is. *That* is the teaching of Tuffel.

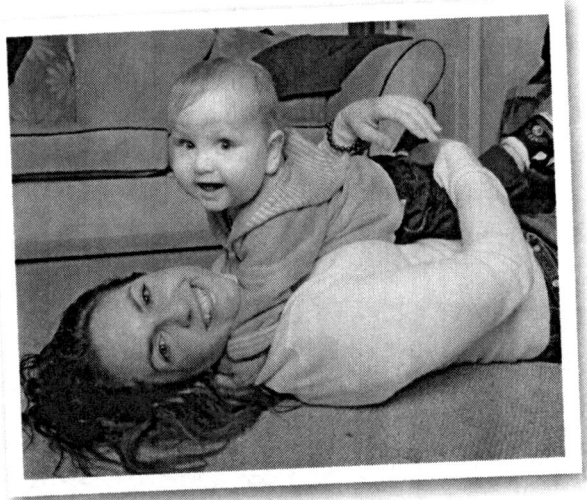

Epilogue

And now?

Tuffel continues to thrive at home. He's been in hospital a fair few times, and on most occasions his high temperatures were due to simple colds or teething issues (he still gets hammered with strong drugs for three days until test results come in) but one was a real line infection, which we luckily caught early.

Tuffel's life is not a given, and wonky liver numbers, which indicate the status of his liver function, keep him on the brink of undergoing biopsies and endoscopies.

Due to the nature of life on artificial nutrition, there's a constant danger of liver damage or contracting dangerous line infections. If these aren't caught early enough, they can turn very nasty. We will continue to live a life of uncertainty, hoping for the best.

However, after much research and connecting with the world's leading scientists, we believe that **there will be a solution for Tuffel** and other children and adults with organ failure. With the help of stem cells, it will be possible to infuse donor organs in order to create rejection-free transplants. And with stem cells, it could be possible to create new organs from scratch. This technology of the future hasn't got enough funding, so we are raising awareness and calling for help!

Just in case you're wondering, this has nothing to do with embryonic stem cells or cloning, or any of the ethically controversial developments you may have heard about. We are talking about the field of regenerative medicine, which is about saving lives. Not cloning it or trying to make 'super humans.' It's about helping humans who have lost vital organs to get a second chance. Humans like you, me and Tuffel. We've teamed up with the world-renowned Great Ormond Street Hospital's Children's Charity to support Dr Paolo De Coppi, the researcher who has already successfully transplanted a stem cell-treated windpipe. He is now working on the small intestine: with your help we could celebrate a major breakthrough in modern medicine in the next five years.

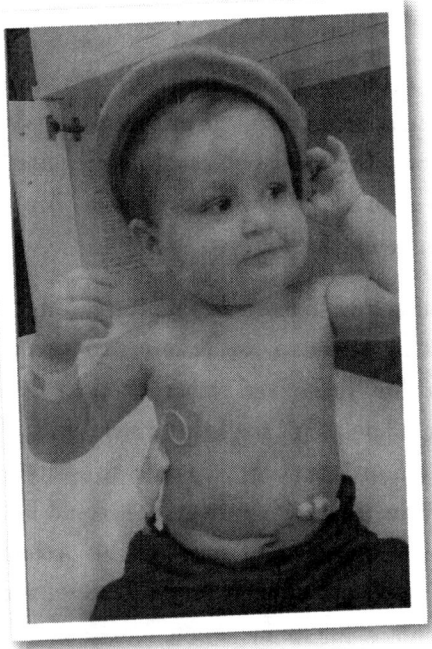

Epilogue

If you are moved by our story and would like to invest in a future in which failing organs are no longer a reason to die, please find out how on www.tuffelstory.com

And please stay in touch with us via Facebook: www.facebook.com/teamtuffel

We appreciate your support deeply.

Evelyne, Thomas and Tuffel

Thank Yous

I want to thank my wonderful editor Selina Altomonte whose dedication went beyond what anyone could ask for. The making of this book is a movie in itself with Selina's first child in intensive care due to a virus, her being in and out of hospital throughout her second pregnancy, giving birth prematurely and juggling two children in and out of medical care units. When her boys were home, mine would be in hospital, or we'd both have our kids on a ward, and thanks to modern technology coordinated much of the editing and adjustments of this book from our bedsides. I've enjoyed the process a lot, though we both had to hold our breath sometimes or, better said, remind each other to breathe in between the calamities.

I want to thank my publishers for their patience. I've missed at least three deadlines. Thankfully they are intelligent women who understood that the author of this book continues to live and juggle the crazy life she's describing. Why am I writing about myself in third person again? I am going mad. Thank you Mindy Gibbins-Klein for publishing me, and thank you to the Panoma Press team (Charlotte and Emma thank you for your kindness and patience and beautiful work)

Thank you Ann Coppens for making the connection to Panoma Press. What a lift this have given me and the creation of the book. Having a great team makes all the difference.

Thank you for your help with checking spelling, Daphne Miles and Sarah-Louise Young.

And Thomas, for your continued encouragement and agreeing to have yourself featured so honestly here. There is, of course, much more to Thomas than you can read in this book! He's a gem of a man.

I want to thank all the people who took time to review the book. Some of you were under great time pressure with your own books and still took the time to read and write for me. Some of you don't write reviews. Some never have. I'm honoured this story moved you so much to do it anyway.

Thank you to Doctor Anthony Kaiser, the longest-standing medic at St Thomas' Neonatal Ward, for writing the foreword and checking medical details for accuracy. And Rich Litvin, my friend and favourite coach, for his foreword too.

To all the nurses, doctors, surgeons and unnamed people who work in hospitals. I think you are amazing. A special thank you to all the unsung heroes of this and countless other stories. Thank you for doing what you do.

Thank you to my long-time mentor and Supercoach Michael Neill for offering to speak when it was most needed and helping me connect to my wellbeing in week 1. My gratitude extends to Robert Holden for your continued support and insights, for being there for me answering some pretty burning questions about karma and love.

I want to thank Lambeth and Greenwich councils for supporting us with care.

I want to say thank you to the NHS. Without the NHS, Tuffel would not be around, or we would be in a very different position. Special care such as Tuffel's is unaffordable to individuals. I am so grateful that our system allows society to pull together to help. The NHS surely has its many challenges, but this experience has let me see it from its best side. And with that I want to thank every tax payer of the United Kingdom for their contribution. I'm glad I opted into NHS contributions when my accountant said I didn't have to. I felt it was important. We are a team making this and other miracles possible. Thank YOU.

Thank you to my wonderful family for being with us and being close when we need it the most. It's not a given. But it has been given. I appreciate all your helping hands, open hearts and loving eyes. The chats, the cuddles, the support. Thank you to my American 'family' for even offering to adopt Tuffel to get him the most advanced care possible, your research, love and ongoing nurturing.

I want to thank you, who are reading this. It's easy to skip the last part where people you may never have heard of get praised. I want to thank you for sharing the journey. Thank you for your thoughts, energy, your spirit. For opening up to your own "possibility thinking". I deeply believe this is how we serve everyone and the planet best.

With love and a twinkle in my eye,

Evelyne

Further Reading

If you'd like to learn more about the groups and associations that have helped us along the way, please see:

PINNT (Patients On Intravenous & Nasogastric Nutrition Therapy) www.pinnt.com

Short Gut Support Forum on Facebook: www.facebook.com/groups/shortgutsupport/

Shooting Stars Children's Hospice: www.shootingstarchase.org.uk

And our story continues, of course – follow our blog at

www.tuffelstory.com

About The Author

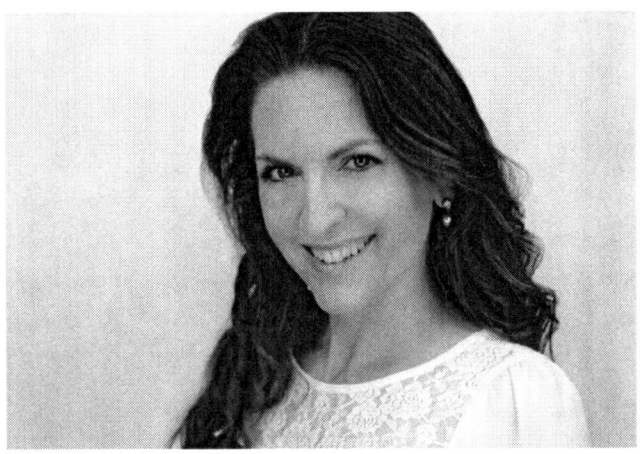

Evelyne Brink is a personal and executive coach, professional speaker and author of "The ARTrepreneur. Financial Success for Artistic Souls" and "The Eye of the Needle", "how to be happy with no easy lessons". She helps committed individuals to shine their light into the world and create from a place of deep aliveness. She has been known as Uk's Nr.1 Madonna impersonator as seen on TV (BBC1, ITV) and has written and produced her own music and shows around the world but many more that never left her head. She loves a laugh, romance and radical honesty. She doesn't actually love the honesty bit when it's personal and painful. She'd prefer having a laugh. In 2012 her partner Thomas and her became parents and her world changed. www.evelynebrink.com

Lightning Source UK Ltd.
Milton Keynes UK
UKOW02f1024201114

241906UK00001B/1/P

9 781909 623729